About the Author:

Shirley Harrison has spent thirty years working in journalism and PR and is now a full-time non-fiction writer. Her most recent book, *The Channel – a historical portrait*, was published in 1986. The book was commissioned as a joint project with her husband, John Harrison, who died of stomach cancer before research began. Three years later Shirley was approached by Donald Stevens of NAC and asked to write a compassionate guide to cancer based on her own understanding of how totally inadequate anyone can feel when confronted with a diagnosis of malignant carcinoma.

NEW APPROACHES TO CANCER

What Everyone Needs to Know About Orthodox and Complementary Methods for Prevention, Treatment and Cure

Shirley Harrison

Preface by Dr Ian Pearce, BA, BM, BCh, MRCS, LRCP
Medical Director, New Approaches to Cancer

CENTURY
LONDON   MELBOURNE   AUCKLAND   JOHANNESBURG

First published in 1987 by Century Hutchinson Ltd,
Brookmount House, 62–65 Chandos Place, Covent Garden,
London WC2N 4NW

Century Hutchinson Australia Pty Ltd,
PO Box 496, 16–22 Church Street, Hawthorn, Victoria 3122,
Australia

Century Hutchinson New Zealand Ltd,
PO Box 40–086, Glenfield, Auckland 10,
New Zealand

Century Hutchinson South Africa Pty Ltd,
PO Box 337, Bergvlei, 2012 South Africa

Reprinted 1987, 1988

British Library Cataloguing in Publication Data

Harrison, Shirley
New approaches to cancer: what everyone needs to
know about orthodox and complementary methods for
prevention, treatment and cure.
1. Cancer
I. Title
616.99'4   RC261
ISBN 0 7126 1488 5

Set in 11/12pt Linotron 202 Sabon
Photoset by Deltatype Lecru, Ellesmere Port, Cheshire
Printed and bound in Great Britain by
Richard Clay Ltd, Bungay, Suffolk

Contents

My journey into the world surrounding cancer has been heartwarming and enriching. The guides who held my hand in hospitals, health centres, laboratories and clinics gave me time and shared their professional knowledge. Patients gave me understanding, opened their hearts and shared their feelings. There has been much humour and less despair than I dared hope. My thanks to them all for their confidence in me — and the future.

I would also like to thank the following individuals and organisations: Dr Linus Pauling; Dr Ian Pearce for permission to quote from *The Gate of Healing* (Jersey Neville Spearman) and for his invaluable help and advice; Penny Brohn for permission to quote from *Gentle Giants* (Century); Beata Bishop for permission to quote an adapted extract from *A Time to Heal* (Severn House); Mikie Sherman for permission to quote from *The Leukaemic Child* (US Dept. of Health); Faber & Faber for permission to quote from *Collected Poems* by W. H. Auden; Methuen Children's Books for permission to quote A. A. Milne; The Society of Authors on behalf of the Bernard Shaw Estate for permission to quote George Bernard Shaw; and the Center for Attitudinal Healing in California for permission to reproduce the illustrations shown on pages 147, 150 and 152 from *There Is A Rainbow Behind Every Dark Cloud*.

Peregrine of Forli

Died 1330. Canonised 1726.
St Peregrine is the Saint invoked for cases of cancer.
He is pictured in 'Saints and their Attributes' as a
penitent, with clasped hands before the Virgin — a
bandage round his leg and foot. He was cured of cancer
of the foot.

Grey are all your theories
Green the growing tree of life
(*Goethe*)

Preface

An Open Letter to the Doctors of Today

Dear Doctor,

'The times they are a-changing.' The medicine which is practised by many of your colleagues is far removed from that practised by my father and in which I was trained. It is no longer the exercise of the art of healing, but has become instead the practice of technological expertise, which is frequently carried out with only superficial consideration of the true best interests of the patient. In its obsession with technology, and its pride in the tremendous advances of the last three decades, it is in danger of forgetting that the true meaning of healing is *making whole*. It has focused its attention upon diseases, to the exclusion of the person manifesting the disease. It has lost its soul!

Nowhere is this clearer than in our attitude to cancer. All too often we concentrate all our efforts upon attempting to eradicate the tumour, frequently by extremely aggressive and unpleasant methods, or upon the alleviation of its effects. Seldom do we ask ourselves '*Why* has this patient developed cancer?' Were we to do so, we would see that the appearance of the tumour is all too often the final stage of a number of processes throughout the patient's life. (We already recognise this in the case of smoking!) This being so, it is futile to attempt to eradicate the tumour without helping to correct the malign influences which provoked it.

Healing is not something which we, in our superior wisdom, do *to* the patient. It is an expression of the force of life, itself divine in essence, within the patient. As such, it is something which the patient does for him or herself. Our task is to cultivate that force, to help to remove the blockages which prevent it from functioning and to maintain life while it is fulfilling its healing function. (This is where technology is necessary. We cannot throw that on one side, but we must always be on our guard that it does not damage the healing force, and so lose more upon the swings than we have gained upon the roundabouts.)

Intuitively, the public is coming to realise this. The time is past when we can give our patients a pat on the head and say 'Doctor knows best!' We have to develop a new relationship – one of partnership – so that they can realise that *they*, too, have a vital role to play.

To do this, we have to be able to communicate – many of us are not very good at this and those within hospitals have tended to leave such matters to our nurses. At long last the art is being taught in medical schools. We often learn the skills of communication from the poor example of over-stressed clinical teachers, or we pick them up as we go along. We make the excuse that we have no time to talk in depth with patients, but the sad truth is that many just do not know where to begin!

Cancer is perhaps the biggest test of our skills. The patient with the diagnosis of cancer believes that he is facing death, that suddenly the future, which seemed so bright, is no longer there. Even though our medical technology has been spectacularly successful with a small number of cancers, the melancholy truth is that one in two patients with breast cancer will die within five years, and that the average survival time with lung cancer remains under two years from the point of diagnosis. Patients know this, and are terrified. In consequence, cancer help services are inundated with requests from desperate people for help which we should be able to give them – and fail.

These figures *can* be improved. But for this to happen it is necessary for us – the doctors – to cast aside our prejudices and to be willing to work with (not upon!) our patients.

You may object that some complementary methods are not scientifically proven; that they do not obey the scientific laws of statistical repetition; that improvements are the consequence of normal therapy, and that new methods are of no more than subjective value. But the evidence to the contrary is there, if you will look for it. At this very moment no less than three trials are taking place to compare the long term effects of a combination of holistic and orthodox therapy with those of orthodox therapy alone. Some of the effects of these new methods, in any case, are not capable of quantification. (How do you quantify joy, happiness, or a sense of fulfilment? How do you measure quality of living, or the route by which any of them are achieved?)

No one is seeking to do away with conventional therapies. But these – *by themselves* – are not enough. They must be complemented by new techniques, and expanded into areas which orthodox medicine does not at present reach. Nutrition, orthomolecular biology, psychotherapy, personal belief and motivation both of patient and therapist, therapeutic touch, prayer and healing all can play a vital part in the healing of cancer.

I beg you to join us. There are innumerable books from which you can learn: seminars and lectures to attend. Even if you feel unable to practise such methods yourself, do at least familiarise yourself with what is happening and give us your cooperation. Get to know, and support, the local complementary professionals, the self-help groups and the national counselling organisations. They can help to lighten your burden, and make life easier, both for you and your patients. To fail in this now may result in the very thing which you least want: that of driving patients away from medicine into the arms of enthusiastic but untrained amateurs. As doctors, we hold the key to every front door in the country. It is an exciting responsibility.

Yours very sincerely,
Ian C. B. Pearce, BA, BM, BCh, MRCS, LRCP
Medical Director, New Approaches to Cancer

1
The Cancer Jungle

There was once an old sailor my grandfather knew
Who had so many things which he wanted to do
That whenever he thought it was time to begin
He couldn't because of the state he was in.

A. A. Milne

It is a familiar feeling. So many choices. So much to do. Which way to turn? Never have we been so bombarded with advice, information and theories on how to live our lives and especially how to stay fit and avoid cancer. For cancer, above all, has become a national obsession. Motor cars, heart disease and alcohol are even more dangerous – but cancer frightens us most.

Jogging is good for you. Jogging is bad. Fibre is in. Fat is out. Milk is a heart stopper. Parsley is carcinogenic, so are parsnips, sex and almost anything else you enjoy. All agree smoking is bad. Plastic bags, nylon tights, sunshine itself, are each on someone's danger list. Everyone is talking about acupuncture but dare you mention it to your doctor? How can you trust a herbalist who says you need Superdofilis at £22 a bottle – or a surgeon who says you need a private operation which might be beneficial to you, but is certainly lucrative to him? Or the hard pressed GP for whom tranquilliser prescriptions still yield the speediest surgery turnover time? What can they, in their turn, do about the 40 per cent of patients who have probably worried their way into the waiting room and should not be there at all?

Human cancers, in particular, seem to thrive in a climate where the need to compete, the removal of taboos, the loss of belief in God or in leaders has become too much for most of us to handle. We flounder. Health has become a religion.

Divorce, bereavement and redundancy probably don't

cause cancers but they are all fuel for them. So, too, are poor, overprocessed food and pollution. So, too, is age, for cancer is one of the natural consequences of ageing and since we all live longer, more of us will get cancer in later life. Many of those dying from cancer in their fifties and sixties today might well have died in their forties or fifties of tuberculosis, then called consumption, a century ago.

In other words, the increase in cancers is probably a reflection of twentieth century lifestyle just as TB was a product of Victorian lack of cleanliness and living conditions. It arises when the cobweb of life is weakened in any one of a hundred places; it strikes princes and paupers alike.

There is no proof as implied in certain television advertisements for the Pharmaceutical Association that TB was conquered by drugs alone. Drugs helped, but the chief credit should go to improvements in sanitation and daily hygiene. Nor is there any proof that drugs alone will kick cancer. There is unlikely ever to be one magic bullet or miracle cure.

Cancer is not an illness which has been superimposed on humanity. It exists in each of us and always has. It was first named by Hippocrates in 420 BC – from the Greek word for a crab, *karkinos* – and is the family name for almost a hundred varieties of disease. It has been found in prehistoric plants and fossils. The conditions we create around it provide the soil on which it grows, and there is a huge element of chance in whether or not it ever gets out of hand in any one of us.

There is little doubt that the key to keeping fit is first to forget about being ill. Don't worry. Granny may well have been right – 'a little of what you fancy does you good'. There are, however, guidelines through the maze which are worth following and which can help you make the best of your lot both when you are well or if you become ill. They apply whether you are breathing carbon monoxide in an inner city or living in rural Wales, whether you are a supercharged executive – or on the dole. Especially important is to adapt any guidelines to your own lifestyle, environment and pocket. It is no good being paranoid about carcinogens in your paint factory if there is no other work in the area. Paranoia is probably as dangerous as paint fumes.

So take heart. Cancer can be an ugly, painful and degrading disease. Frequently, it is none of these. Remember there is no such thing as cancer of the spirit.

The statistics are bad, so turn statistics on their head. Twenty-nine per cent of us gets cancer. One in five dies of it. That means four out of five survives with – or without. Everywhere you look, on the escalators, on the buses, down at the supermarket, there are people – shopping, travelling, living, with cancer. You would never know. It is not always the immediate, relentless killer we dread. So many of those in whom, for one reason or another, cancer breaks out, carry on regardless. Why has there been so little study into the causes of survival?

Bob Champion rode in the Grand National after being told he had cancer. Sir Francis Chichester sailed solo round the world with lung cancer. Solzhenitsyn, who wrote *Cancer Ward*, was diagnosed in his mid-fifties and then went on to marry and have two children. Sigmund Freud had mouth cancer when 60 and died in his eighties.

In the end, should your cancer surface, only you can decide what to do about it. The danger with the discovery that the future is, to a degree, your responsibility, is the inevitable sense of guilt should things work out badly. But cancer is a capricious, baffling disease. You can't pin-point exactly why you get it. Nor can you be sure why one person dies and another lives. There is no blame. The only certainty is that hopes are much greater for optimistic lovers of life who try to banish all negative thoughts and get on with the job of living – both with and without cancer.

Of course, medicine has made tremendous strides in the care of this twentieth-century 'roller coaster', but in so doing we have lost track of the truth that good health comes only with a balance of healthy mind, body and spirit. With trust and teamwork today, the old order is changing. In the last five years there has been a mushrooming of natural health clinics and cancer self-help groups all over Britain. On the one hand, there has never been so much understanding community help, backed by caring, if overstretched, medical services: on the other, so much confusion.

The aim of this book is to guide you through unfamiliar and scary country. Not to tell you how to travel – but the choices you may meet, so that you can seek more detailed expert advice when you find a route that feels right for you. It is written, too, for the 'armchair' traveller who is seeing cancer from afar with no personal experience. You may never find yourself plunged into this jungle, confronted with such danger; but the jungle is all around, tapping at the window. By being prepared you may keep it from breaking in.

The book looks purposely on the brighter side, because therein lies the key to success; also with realism, for it would be wrong to ignore facts we all experience. We know that NHS patients face appalling hospital waiting lists and often cavalier treatment from consultants who have learned to view illness as a mechanical breakdown and seem lacking in compassion and humanity. We know that in orthodox medicine mistakes are all too often made and on the other hand, we are aware that complementary therapies and medicine can be expensive.

Today, once cancer is diagnosed, you can choose to hit the thing head on with the benefits of science through chemotherapy, radiotherapy, surgery, or you may take such gentler complementary routes as acupuncture, psychotherapy or diet. Or – so important – you may use both. That is your right and there is a better chance of achieving this ideal than at any time this century.

Neither traditional nor complementary approaches has a monopoly over your health. They should be pulling together, with the aim of making you well. The choice on offer should not be 'either/or', always 'both/and' – and because they are so much in the public mind those working with cancer could carry the flag of cooperation for the medical world as a whole.

Remember, the Chinese symbol for crisis contains the symbols for both danger and opportunity. That's life. That's cancer.

Contrary to Nature

Each gram of human tissue contains about 100,000,000 cells. (One level teaspoonful of sugar weighs 5 grams.) A baby begins from just one cell, formed from the fusion of a female egg and male sperm. This multiplies until there are about 60 trillion cells adapted to tackle the making of different organs and tissues. It is believed that these are constantly renewed so that within every seven years we are completely 'new' people, made up of vigorous new cells.

When all is well

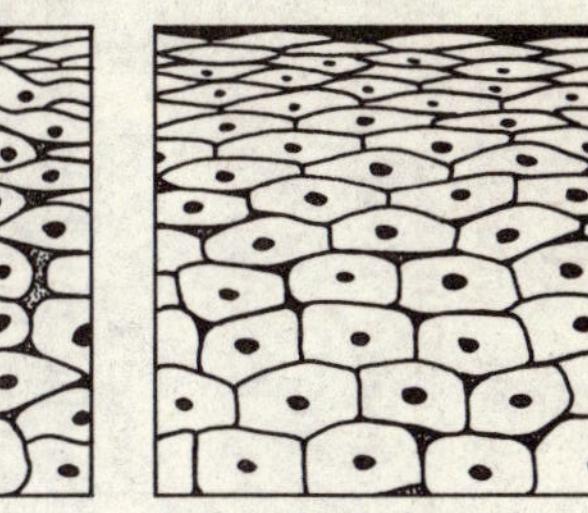

1. Microscopic selection from your 10 million million cells.

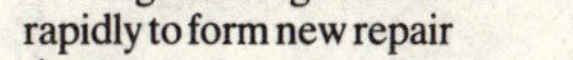

2. Damage caused, perhaps by cut.

3. Neighbouring cells divide rapidly to form new repair tissue.

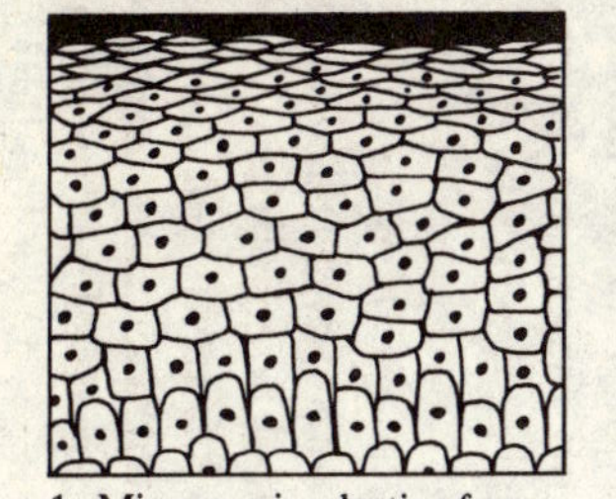

4. Once healed, steady maintenance routine continuously replaces dead cells.

When this goes wrong

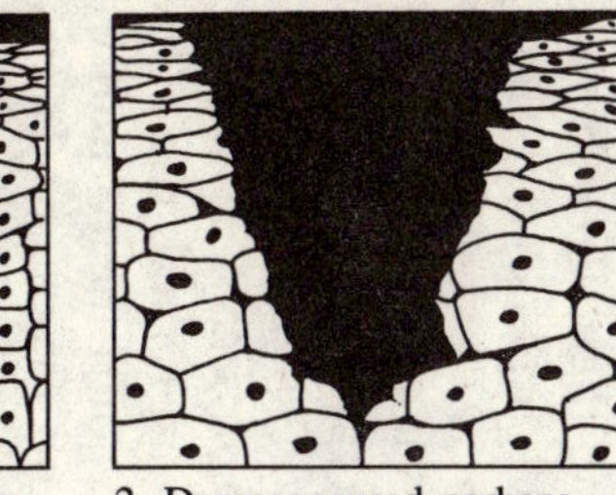

1. Occasionally there is a fault and one cell gives the wrong reproductive signal.

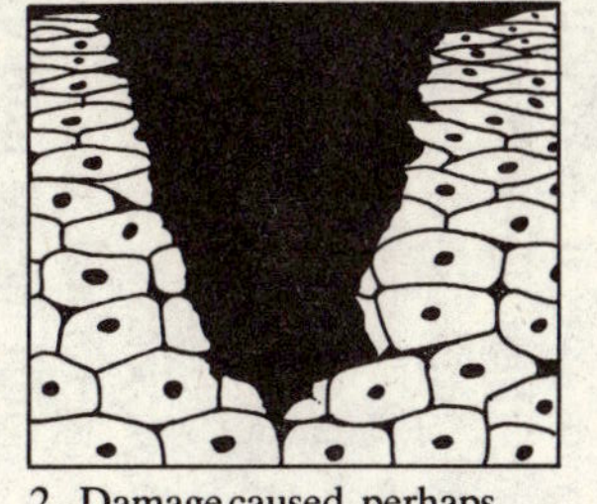

2. It begins uncontrolled dividing and formation of a mass which is not part of the original organ or tissue. This mass grows and prevents their correct functioning. This is called local invasion.

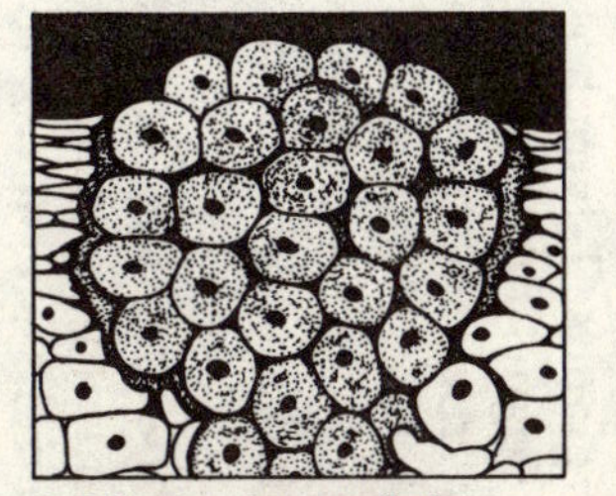

3. Sometimes one of these cells may break off and travel through the body to form new colonies. This is a secondary growth – metastases.

The process is largely controlled by what scientists call DNA (Deoxyribonucleic Acid), a molecule which is the basic chemical blueprint for the creation of new cells. It is the computer programme for each cell. How the programme is designed is the mystery. DNA is the raw material of life and it is found throughout the living world, from amoebas to man.

Sometimes – and no one knows why – the DNA fails to tell the cell to stop dividing at the right time and it runs amok. Like a rogue elephant, it gets out of control.

About 100,000 malignant cells are present in each of us every day. They are probably destroyed by the immune system which is believed to defend the body by attacking intruders. This is known as 'surveillance theory'.

What is the Immune System?

Our understanding of the immune system is a grey area. Its functioning is a mystery still. Every chemical intruder bears a fingerprint – known as the antigen – which identifies it and warns the body of a threat. In some cases the white cells from the thymus glands (T-lymphocytes) produce an army of killers to destroy rogue intruders by dissolving them. In others it is white cells from the bone marrow (B-lymphocytes) that go into battle. The resulting debris is then cleared up by the macrophages – the body's vacuum cleaners (cells which recognise and attack waste or faulty organisms).

What Happens when Cancer Runs Amok?

When the immune system is weak or suppressed, the aggressive cancer cells are uncontrolled and continue to multiply. They take up more and more room and invade body tissue preventing its proper function. Why they take off in the first place is the great unknown.

There are many theories. Some say there is a genetic weakness inherited at birth from father or mother (they say we don't inherit cancer – we do inherit a weakened ability to deal with it). Some believe it may be due to chemicals released as a reaction to physical or mental stress, others that pollution from food and the atmosphere are the culprits. The newest line of research is the attempt to identify a virus. Most likely it is a combination of any – or all – of these.

Because the original rogue cell can originate in any part of

the body there are over a hundred different forms of cancer.
These are some of the forms and the parts affected:

Melanomas	The skin
Carcinomas	The skin or organ linings
Sarcomas	Muscle or bone
Leukaemias	Blood
Lymphomas	The lymph glands

Some cancers develop very slowly, lying dormant for 20 or 30
years. Some may grow like a balloon. Others spread like lava.
They can be mushy or fibrous, prefer the old or the young, the
Iranians or the Germans, asbestos workers or Japanese
fishermen. There can be different kinds of cancer within the
same organ. Generally nature seems to balance itself out, for
where in one country you find a high incidence of one cancer
there will be low incidences of the rest.

Very often the malignant cells break away from their
original site and form new colonies of abnormal cells. These
secondary growths are called metastases and are the most
lethal problem of all, because they can settle in vital organs
such as the brain and lung.

Lymphatic spread The lymph system is the network of vessels
throughout the body, designed to remove impurities via the
lymph nodes, which act as filters. If the roving cancer cells get
trapped in the nodes this system is blocked and the network
becomes a transmitter of malignancy.

Bloodstream spread If the cancer cells invade the bloodstream,
again they may be carried anywhere. The major site to which
bowel cancer spreads, for instance, is the liver because the
veins draining the bowel pass blood to the liver.

The Cancer Business

The disease of cancer will be banished from life by calm
unhurrying persistent men and women working with every shiver
of feeling controlled and suppressed in hospitals and laboratories
and the motive that will conquer cancer will not be pity nor
horror. It will be curiosity to know how and why.

H. G. Wells

Perhaps the prose of H. G. Wells should be offset against the poetry of A. A. Milne.

> No one can tell me,
> Nobody knows,
> Where the wind comes from,
> Where the wind goes.

A. A. Milne

Since the foundation of Britain's longest established research institute – the Imperial Cancer Research Fund – in 1902, similar organisations have developed in every civilised country. Cancer has become a major, expanding employer of hundreds of thousands of people worldwide: in most western countries, more people are employed in the cancer business than die of the disease. Tremendous strides have been made in our accumulated knowledge of cancer. Oncology, the study of tumours, has become a profession in its own right. Yet, despite research expenditure of over £20bn in the last 20 years, there is almost no change in the proportion of those who live or die. Science has discovered what happens when cancer begins – not *why* it begins. In America, for instance, less than 2 per cent of the National Cancer Research budget is dedicated to prevention, the rest to cure. Cancer remains mockingly remote – and intact.

'The course of cancer is as unpredictable as the individual. Having formed, it may not grow; having grown, it may not disease or trouble; having diseased, it may not kill.' So say Drs Kothari and Mehtha in *Cancer, the Realities of Cause and Cure*. It is indeed like looking for the meaning of life.

So why bother? The author of *The Siege of Cancer*, scientist Dr June Goodfield says:

> We guarantee neither total eradication nor total cure. Even if we did find a cure, the increase in life expectancy would be minute. The vast sums of money that would be required are, on the face of it, out of all proportion to the statistics. . . . So what is the rationale? To pose the question in such cold blooded terms is to ignore the haunting dimension of cancer – the human being. Sometimes arguments have to be made on compassion and compassion alone.

Even so, there are many medical people who feel cancer is over-funded and over-researched. They believe that work starts one rung too far up the ladder and that much more could be researched into the cancer personality – the soil in which it grows. In 1984, the Cancer Research Campaign and the Imperial Cancer Research Fund alone were fourth and fifth in the grant-seeking charities league – with a total of £38,000,000 voluntary income, compared with, say, £6,691,000 to the British Heart Foundation for a disease that kills more people. Only Oxfam, the National Trust and the Royal National Lifeboat Institution are up in front.

Twice Nobel prize winner for chemistry, Dr Linus Pauling of the American Institute of Science and Medicine, has even claimed that 'most cancer research is a fraud and the major cancer research organisations are derelict in their duties to the people who support them.'

According to Samuel Epstein in *The Politics of Cancer*, it is not a scientific problem at all. It is political. In 1960, the World Health Organisation estimated that 60–70 per cent of cancers are caused by diet and lifestyle and therefore preventable – were it not that all the things which can trigger cancer represent huge profitable vested interests.

Percentage of Cancer Patients Diagnosed in 1975 Who Were Still Alive in 1980

Type of Cancer	Women	Men
Uterus	65.8	
Skin (malignant melanoma)	66.4	52.4
Breast	57.4	
Lymph (Hodgkin's)	52.9	58.2
Cervical	51.7	
Bladder	47.8	54.2
Lymph (general)	37.1	40.5
Prostate		35.1
Kidney	31.2	31.3
Rectum	30.6	30.6
Colon	29.5	31.3
Ovary	23.5	
Leukaemia	18.1	18.0
Oesophagus	8.1	5.6
Stomach	7.4	6.9
Lung	6.6	7.0
Pancreas	3.6	2.8

From: 'Observer', 17 August 1986.

In the Charities Aid Foundation *Directory of Cancer Research and Welfare Organisations*, dozens of worthy bodies are listed in all parts of Britain. It would be utterly mistaken to wipe them off the slate. There is so much excellent work in progress. The point at issue is emphasis – perhaps too much on cure and not enough on prevention, too much on why patients die and not why they live.

The Dimbleby Factor

In November 1965 an announcement appeared in the Press. It had been written by David Dimbleby at the request of his father, the much beloved 'voice of Britain', Richard Dimbleby.

> My father first contracted cancer five years ago and has been undergoing treatment at various times since then. He has asked me to explain this because he is very strongly opposed to the idea of cancer being an unmentionable disease. The reason he has not mentioned it is that he has not lost a single day's work, but as he expects to be away for a few weeks he thought that people ought to know why.

That simple statement was hailed as a courageous act. The *Daily Mirror* said: 'Richard Dimbleby . . . has broken one of the greatest taboos of this century. Cancer is an unmentionable subject. Until a few days ago no popular paper would even print the word . . . We should be able to talk about cancer as we talk about measles.'

Seven thousand letters poured in, expressing thanks and, most of all, a sense of tremendous relief that a personality as famous as Richard Dimbleby had shared his suffering. Cancer patients felt they were not alone. This was the first time that a public figure had spoken honestly. It marked a watershed in the story of a disease that had previously not even been identified on death certificates.

Figureheads can be a tremendous influence for good or bad. Richard Dimbleby was revered in those post-war years in a way no other man apart from Churchill had been. His honest dignity was an inspiration. What the public did not know was how Richard had given similar strength to his family – the children, David, Jonathan, Sally and Nicholas, and wife, Dilys – and how from the very beginning they had supported each other and pulled together as a team. 'We learned to live with it,' recalls Jonathan. 'My mother never had to make excuses if he became tired or irritable and he didn't have to carry the secret.'

Jonathan's moving biography of his father helped to change public attitudes. He revealed the phenomenal work load cheerfully undertaken by Richard Dimbleby at the peak of his profession at the same time as grappling with a painful and insidiously debilitating cancer. His diary is proof of what can be done. In the period 26 April to 14 June

> he had done more than twenty major programmes; he had made ten European and four transatlantic flights; he had endured five serious radiotherapy sessions, and an operation for the removal of a malignant tumour from his scalp.
>
> The next month was spent attempting to halt a cancer which had spread throughout his body and now extended from his groin to his scalp. Between the middle of June and the month of July he went to hospital nineteen times for radiotherapy and was given forty-three treatments to his abdomen, neck, scalp, ribs, spine, shoulders and lymphatic glands. Throughout the month, he continued to introduce *Panorama*.

When Richard Dimbleby died on 22 December 1965, the family were overwhelmed by the public's distress. Instead of flowers a fund was established to help cancer treatment, especially at St Thomas's Hospital, London. Today the Richard Dimbleby Fund, which is still administered by the family, donates money not only for research but for care groups, day centres, hospices, spiritual and alternative therapies. 'We try to help lesser known organisations without famous names.'

2
The Cancer Story

There are two fundamentally different ways of looking at health. In the past they have been uneasy bedfellows.

Cartesian philosophy is named after the eighteenth century Frenchman, Réné Descartes, who believed in the sharp division of body and soul. He claimed the body, being ruled by mechanical laws, should be treated separately from the soul, which is immortal. It is on Cartesian ideas – 'The whole is the sum of its parts' – that modern western medicine is based. Medical students are still taught to see the body as a collection of cells and organs and to disbelieve anything that cannot be proved. This is why there is such resistance to any medical theory which is not, by its nature, scientifically quantifiable – such as homoeopathy or healing.

Holistic belief is that mind, body and spirit cannot be separated: 'The whole is *greater* than the sum of its parts.' You cannot, therefore, treat physical sickness without considering the whole being. So, because holistic therapies recognise the mental, emotional and spiritual aspects of the person as well as the physical, they cannot be subjected to the kind of clinical tests that the medical profession demands as proof.

Humans are deaf to the sound a bat hears. We can't see radio waves, yet we can listen to *Top of the Pops*. How does a man walking on burning coals escape unscathed? How does acupuncture replace anaesthetic? Think on these things and it makes sense that there is more to the body than its working, that there are some questions to which as yet there are no answers. Most GPs admit that tender loving care works more miracles than tranquillisers.

There is nothing new in the rift between these approaches. It began two and a half thousand years ago with Hippocrates, the ancient Greek upon whose name newly qualified medical students once swore 'to do no harm'. Hippocrates was the first and perhaps the greatest naturopath; he used natural remedies, herbs and diet. Only after his death did his followers over-emphasise the scientific aspects of his teaching and move away from nature in medicine. They swung so far, in fact, that by 380 BC Plato was provoked into an outburst in which he declared

> The cure of the part should not be attempted without the treatment of the whole. No attempt should be made to cure the body without the soul and if the head and body are to be healthy you must begin by curing the mind.

The Jews had a very different attitude. Healing was in the hands of the priests and if you didn't get better it was divine retribution. No wonder the arrival of Jesus upset them. He commanded his disciples to preach the gospel *and* heal the sick. He Himself used every possible form of healing from absent healing to the laying on of hands.

For hundreds of years after the death of Jesus, healing and preaching were the cornerstones of Christianity. Not till the Middle Ages, when priests became more concerned with intellectual affairs and power, did the Church's healing role decline and healers become ranked with witches. Blood letting was banned and surgery was practised only by barbers outside the Church.

Dominating the entire period from about 200 AD to the Renaissance was the medical influence of the great Galen, who believed, like Hippocrates, that cancer was due to an excess of black bile and best left alone.

As knowledge increased, the gap widened. Scientific medicine became confined to a small group of secular academics whilst holism was instinctively understood and practised by the masses. Every village had its priest and its wise woman. Physicians were to be found only in great cities.

Finally, in the nineteenth century, a medical revolution jettisoned the intuitive wisdom of some three thousand years. With improved equipment and better hygiene, scientific medicine became 'orthodox' and anything else was 'on the fringe'. Doctors became intoxicated with their new power and rightly proud of their skill. They forgot such simple truths that everyone's Granny knew . . . that if you, for instance, filled a well-worn, unwashed sock with cooking salt and heated it in the oven and then tied it round the patient's neck, minor throat ailments would vanish!

Since then we have learned, without question, to apply the word orthodox to the work of the GP, the hospital, the surgeon and the nurse. Anyone practising in any other approach is regarded as 'alternative' or 'complementary'. We forgot that, worldwide, acupuncture, herbalism and healing had been woven into man's history. It is only in the last 150 years that the impressive might of mechanistic medicine has claimed a total monopoly of health care in the west.

Ironically, it is conventional medicine which is complementary. Grasp hold of that idea and there is better hope of ultimately breaking the magic circle, so that experts in all disciplines may at long last work side by side, for none is all-embracing, each has validity.

For wise men and women there are, in every branch of healing, and wisdom there is, too, in every one of us, if we have the confidence to trust ourselves. This time, that confidence seems to be arising through widespread public dissatisfaction with the established order. Time for a *change*.

In 1986, the British Holistic Medical Association organised its first conference attended by doctors and the lay public. Today, some hospitals run seminars to which BHMA members are invited and there are a number of joint research projects underway.

The twentieth century thirst for scientific knowledge has provoked a tidal wave of research far too complex to catalogue here. But a cure for cancer has, undoubtedly, become the Holy Grail.

In 1947, the National Health Service was founded in Britain and the World Health Organisation in Geneva; each has played its part in the quest. The development of microbiology, virus vaccines and chemotherapy are woven into the story, and every week newspapers announce some new discovery, a new mirage maybe, to bring sometimes hope, sometimes confusion to us all.

We are living through immense social and cultural upheaval, which is affecting attitudes to medicine and which lies behind public dissatisfaction with the established order. Fritjof Capra says in his thought-provoking book *The*

Medicine and Cancer: A Genealogical Table up to the Twentieth Century

The Development of Medicine

Sumerian Medical knowledge based on astronomy. The blood regarded as the source of every vital function, and liver as the collecting centre and so the seat of life.

Babylonian Understood the role played by insects and animals in the spread of disease. It was 'not lawful to pass a sick man by in silence without taking an interest in his complaint' said the Greek historian Herodotus.

The Egyptians Understood the medical use of many drugs, including opium and hemlock. They believed that the heart was the centre of circulation but supposed that this depended on breathing. They founded the first national health service, doctors being paid by the state. In wartime and on journeys anywhere in Egypt the sick were treated free. Physicians specialised for the first time: the tomb of one Dr Iry – around 2,500 BC – states he was 'keeper of the King's rectum'.

Events Relating to Cancer

Evidence that cancer had been established by this period for millions of years in that traces of the disease have been found in dinosaur fossils.

5,000
BC

Cancer found in mummies.
'If thou examinest a man having bulging tumours on his breast and thou findest that swellings have spread over the breast . . . and thou findest them very cool, there being no fever . . . they have no granulation, they form no fluid, they do not generate secretions of fluid . . . there is no treatment.' Egyptian papyrus.

Imhotep, court magician, earliest named healer: his symbol was a snake and he became a demi-god. **2,900 BC**

Ancient India Pioneers in the use of plastic surgery. Rhinoplasty (reconstruction after the nose had been cut off as a punishment for adultery) was commonly performed. They knew that a successful graft had to come from the patient's body. Brahmin influence called for strict hygiene, vegetarian diet and no alcohol. **3,000 BC 2,000**

Caustic arsenic ointment used to treat breast tumours – a form of chemotherapy! First recorded diagnosis of cancer in the epic *Ramayana*.

The Chinese The Emperor, Shen Nung, compiles a herbal which is much the same as today's. They also introduce smallpox immunisation and appreciated the importance of the pulse. Acupuncture was standard medicine. **2,838**

The Jews Became leaders in the concept of disease prevention. In addition to cleanliness and health regulations, they instigated the 'day of rest' . . . to the benefit of all mankind.

Jesus established healing as part of Christian teaching – the laying on of hands, power of prayer, use of spittle.

The Greeks The god of medicine – Asklepios – rose from the Greek interpretation of the stories of Imhotep. His daughter, Hygeia, was goddess of health. Patients slept overnight in his temples, and priests treated them according to their dreams. The practice ceased with the increase in medical knowledge and rise of secular physicians.

Hippocrates, first secular and holistic physician, founder of modern medicine, born on Kos. He defined the doctor's ethics still in use today. Considered that personality is the physician and medicine provides only symptomatic relief. Did not believe in the religious rituals of healing, astrology.

460 BC Cancer is named by Hippocrates from the Greek word for crab – *karkinos*. He made the distinction between superficial and concealed cancer and warned that surgery could worsen the latter.

The birth of Christ.

Galen born in Pergamon (Turkey) was the medical authority of the west for 1,500 years. Wrote 400 books. Took Greek medicine to Rome.

38 AD Galen writes a book on tumours and says they are contrary to nature. Instigates the belief that excessive black bile is the cause of cancer. From *melan cholos*, the Greek words for 'black bile' comes our word 'melancholy'.

Celsus writes *de Medicina* – the greatest Latin work on medicine – the bridge between Hippocrates and Galen.	1st century	Book V of *de Medicina* concerned with cancer. Detailed descriptions and remedies but says there is no cure.
Queen Radegund. First authentic woman doctor. Founds hospital at Poitiers.	570	
Islamic Medicine Avicenna writes Canon of Medicine. Preferred cautery to surgery. Abulkasim – the only important Arab surgeon – used a red hot poker.	980–1037	Wrote poetically of the differences between cancerous swelling and induration, described as 'a slumbering silent mass' – a non-malignant tumour.
	1150	Avenzoar of Cordoba suggests nutrient enemas and special diets for stomach and oesophagus cancer.
Mediaeval Period First medical schools founded in Europe.	10th & 11th centuries	
Medicine and surgery separated when blood letting by clerics was banned by the church. It became relegated to barbers who shaved and bled. Medicine was a blend of astrology, herbs, purgation. The church condemns those who practise without its blessing and healing becomes a 'maverick art'.	12th century	

Healing as practised by Jesus regarded as akin to witchcraft. Development of science and medicine encourages non-clerics to become physicians.	1267	Theodoric of Sienna writes 'The older a cancer is the worse it is. And the more it is involved with muscles, veins and nutrifying arteries the worse it is & more difficult to treat . . . but if the cancer should be in the fleshy places . . . incise it as far as the sound flesh and burn it away afterwards.'
John of Arderne, first great surgeon of England, wrote personal case histories of patients and was a specialist in the medical problems of knights on horseback.	1307–1390	Describes cancer of the rectum: 'Bubo (cancer) is an apostem [festering] breeding within the anus in the rectum with great hardness but little aching . . . to that also will leeches . . . assure the patient that he has dysentery, that is, the bloody flux, when truly it is not . . . dysentery is always with flux of the intestines but out of bubo goes hard excretions and some times they may not pass because of the constriction caused by the bubo so that they may be felt with the finger and drawn out.'
Renaissance Gutenburg's invention of moveable type had far reaching effects on the spread of medical knowledge.	1500	
Paracelsus burns the books of Avicenna and Galen and breaks with the medical past.		The study of oncology at a standstill.

De Humani Corporis Fabrica by Vesalius – a superb study of the human body leads to the development of the study of anatomy. This was the birth of modern medicine. **1543**

Johannes and Zacharia Jansen (Holland) invent microscope. **1590**

Invention of the WC by John Harington, who wrote *The Metamorphosis of Ajax* – a humorous illustrated manual. **1596**

17th century The birth of experimental medicine. Leeuwenhoek explores with microscopes and confirms Harvey's theory of blood circulation.

Gasparo Aselli discovers the lymphatic system. **1581–1627**

Dr Thomas Sydenham – the 'English Hippocrates' – encourages doctors to study their patients, not text books. **1624–1689** Galen's black bile theory ousted, and lymph node removal became common treatment. The belief that cancer is contagious first appears.

Hermann Boerhaave re-established clinical teaching in medicine. **1668–1738**

18th century Study of morbid anatomy and physiology develops.	1700	The first systematic study of carcinogenic environments – *De Morbis Artificium*.
	1703	Ramagini notes that breast cancer incidence is high in nuns, low in wet nurses! Discussion of cancer as a hereditary disease. Patients often refused admission to hospital. Theory of causal inflammation.
Morgagni – the founder of pathology.	1682–1771	
Lind establishes efficacy of citrus fruits to treat scurvy, continuing the findings of Sir Riched Hawkins, 1716–1794, 100 years before vitamin deficiencies understood.		
Benjamin Franklin in the USA invents bifocal spectacles.	1706–1790	
	1740	First specialist cancer hospital founded in Rheims. Then moved due to public pressure and fear of epidemic.
John Hunter, father of scientific surgery, anatomy, dentistry and obstetrics.	1728–1793	
	1761	John Hills cautions against the Immoderate Use of Snuff, as a possible cause of cancer.

| 1775 | First recorded use of experimental animal – Peyrilhe injects human cancer into a dog. Percivall Pott, surgeon at St Bartholomew's Hospital, London, becomes first source of knowledge about chemical carcinogens. He declares cancer of the scrotum a result of exposure to soot. |

Franz Anton Mesmer – the foundation of the theory of animal magnetism and hypnotherapy. — 1734–1815

Joseph Priestley discovers nitrous oxide – analgesic gas. — 1772

Edward Jenner vaccinates labourers with matter from cowpox sores to avoid smallpox. — 1749–1823

| 1792 | 12 bed ward opens for cancer cases at the Middlesex Hospital, funded by Samuel Whitbread. The Middlesex Hospital Cancer Charity – the first cancer institute in the world. |

The publication of *The Morbid Anatomy of Some of the Most Important Parts of the Human Body*. — 1793

Samuel Frederick Hahnemann develops 'like cures like' – theory of homoeopathy. — 1755–1843

Astley Paston Cooper pioneers vascular and testicular surgery. — 1768–1841

19th century The flowering of invention changes the face of medicine too: Pasteur, scientific medicine, the thermometer, anaesthetics, the discovery of X-rays, radiation and genetics, chemotherapy.

The first surgery on internal cancers. Specific cancers identified all through century.

	1801	Institution for Investigating the Nature and Cure of Cancer formed.
Réné Theophile Hyacinthe Laennec discovers the stethoscope.	1781–1826	
Hickman Henry Hill uses carbon dioxide on an animal amputation.	1824	
Microscopes manufactured in London and Paris.	1825+	
	1829	Recamier recognises how cancer spreads and names metastases.
	1832	Hodgkin's Disease named after Professor Thomas Hodgkins.
First use of thermometer for scientific measurement of human body temperatures.	1835	
First use of ether by Sir James Simpson.	1837	First book on tumours published in the USA.
Beginnings of statistics and epidemiology.	1830–1840	

Ignaz Semmelweiss makes students wash hands – puerperal fever declines! Development of anti-sepsis.	1840s	
	1844	Multiple myeloma identified by Henry Bence Jones.
	1845	John Hughes Bennet in Scotland and Rudolf Virchow in Germany identify leukaemia.
Ether used in Massachusetts General Hospital.	1846	
Sir James Simpson uses chloroform.	1811–1870	
Queen Victoria gives birth to Prince Leopold under chloroform.	1847	
The First Public Health Act.	1848	
Florence Nightingale in the Crimea.	1854	
Cholera checked, John Snow tracing infection to contaminated drinking water.	1854	
Virchow develops cellular pathology.	1858	
Charles Darwin's *Origin of the Species*.	1859	
John Hughlings Jackson founds neurology.	1860	
Lord Lister develops asepsis.	1861	

1862	Formation of the Red Cross.
1867	Christian Albert Theodor Billröth – surgical giant working in Vienna.
1870	Moriz Kaposi identifies Kaposi's Sarcoma.
1871	Resection of the oesophagus.
1873	Excision of the larynx.
1881	Partial gastrectomy.
1895	X-rays discovered by Wilhelm Roentgen.
1899	Wilms' tumour named after Max Wilms.
1900	Paul Ehrlich introduces chemotherapy.
1902	Hormone treatment used for the first time.

Turning Point, 'What we need, to prepare ourselves for the great transition we are about to enter, is a deep re-examination of the main values of our culture, a rejection of those models that have outlived their usefulness, and a new recognition of some of those values discarded in previous periods.'

This is also true of medicine and the story of cancer. Today, international communication puts us in easy touch with a vast range of medical knowledge, from the simple tribal remedies of Amazonian Indians, to the spiritual awareness of the east and the sophisticated techniques of the world's great cancer hospitals. Because life and history move in cycles we should not forget the past or the primitive but learn to cherish accumulated wisdom.

3
Life Without Cancer

'The body of man contains in itself blood, phlegm, yellow bile and black bile, which are things in the natural constitution of his body, and the cause of sickness and of health. He is healthy when they are in proper proportion between one another as regards mixture, force and quantity, and when they are well mingled together; he becomes sick when one of these is diminished or increased in amount or separated in the body from its proper mixture and not properly mingled with all the others . . .'

The Four Humours from The Nature of Man

Balance – A Plea from Prince Charles

Don't overestimate the 'sophisticated' approach to medicine. Please don't underestimate the importance of an awareness of what lies beneath the surface of the visible world and of those ancient, unconscious forces which still help to shape the psychological attitudes of modern man. Sophistication is only skin deep and when it comes to healing people it seems to me that account has to be taken of those sometimes long neglected complementary methods of medicine which, in the right hands, can bring considerable relief if not hope to an increasing number of people. I hope that, while maintaining and improving the standards with which the Association is so rightly concerned, the medical profession will at the same time keep a corner of its mind open enough to admit those shafts of light which can preserve a sense of paradox so vital to our sense of unity with nature.

Prince Charles to the BMA, 29 June 1983

Sadly, they didn't listen. In July 1986 the BMA published a report on alternative medicine. Not one alternative specialist was consulted. It said:

When theory and methodology fail it is time for honesty. In fairness to the practitioners of alternative medicine, it has to be said that many patients are comforted, and may be 'healed', when under their care. It is also possible that among the multiplicity of techniques there are some which are genuinely therapeutic, even beyond any placebo effect. Careful study of this possibility is needed, with a view to bringing beneficial techniques within the safeguards offered by a registered profession.

There is, however, another side to the problem. While we have a duty of fairness to the practitioners of alternative therapies, our long-term duty to our patients is not to support what may be passing fashions, but to ensure for them the benefits of medicine in the future. These include future applications of scientific knowledge; but also, and just as important, orthodox medicine carries the safeguards which arise from entrusting the preservation of health and the care of disease to a registered, recognised and accountable profession, with a long-standing tradition of scientific and personal integrity, including strict standards of confidentiality.

Yin and Yang

Under heaven all can see beauty only as beauty because there is
   ugliness.
All can know good as good only because there is evil.
Therefore having and not having arise together.
Difficult and easy complement each other.
Long and short contrast each other;
High and low rest upon each other;
Voice and sound harmonise each other;
Front and back follow one another;
Therefore the sage goes about doing nothing, teaching no talking.
The ten thousand things rise and fall without cease
Creating, yet not possessing,
Working, yet not taking credit.
Work is done, then forgotten.
Therefore it lasts for ever.

'Balance' from the 'Tao Te Ching'

The Chinese have always seen life as an interplay between two interconnected forms of energy – Yin and Yang – sometimes described as the 'shady side and the sunny side of the mountain'. The sunny side – the Yang – is positive, active, physical, scientific, masculine, hot. The Yin is negative, receptive, cool, thoughtful, intuitive, feminine. Everything is either *Yin* or *Yang* and the ideal is to achieve perfect balance. It is a nebulous concept and hard for the western mind to embrace. There is an ancient text which says 'The Yin having reached its climax retreats in favour of the Yang. The Yang having reached its climax retreats in favour of the Yin.'

There is no Chinese word for cancer – it is 'an invasion of cold dampness' and so, statistically, does not exist.

For the last 600 years, western society has, they say, been pursuing a Yang course – active rather than contemplative, scientific rather than religious, belligerent rather than pacific. But there are changes. The Yang is retreating and, as it does so, our male-dominated society is seeing an increasing feminine awareness. There is a pronounced concern with mysticism, a growing interest in holistic health and a return to healing – even in religious circles which have for so long frowned on such 'occult' activity.

For instance, a few medical schools and the Royal College of Nursing include rudimentary acupuncture and holistic health care in their syllabus. Doctors use hypnosis. Orthopaedic surgeons venture to recommend osteopathy; it is a beginning. More and more GPs are converting. True, there are still many hostile hospitals with no counselling services who will not even put the local self-help group posters on their notice boards for fear of upsetting patients; true, canteens still sell over-cooked, over-salted or over-sweetened food. There was no holistic contributor to the 1986 *Which* report on alternative medicine.

There is a grass roots movement coming from a telly-taught people, disillusioned with the 'whip it out quick' tactics of the last hundred years. Being better informed, we are looking to ways in which we can side-step cancer simply by taking more care of ourselves. According to one Norfolk family doctor, the public will 'drag their doctors with them screaming and kicking into the twentieth century.'

The signs are more encouraging than they have ever been.

Food the Fuel – Nutrition

It is common sense that what you put into your body must affect its performance. This applies whether or not you have cancer. There is no need to go over the top on nutrition or to feel guilty about drooling over a bacon 'butty'. There *is* a need to understand what we are eating, how it is grown and, where possible, how, in the long run to avoid gumming up the works. A sound diet is not itself a guarantee of perfect health but it is a step in the right direction and, most important, it is something you *can* control.

Authorities of all kinds, especially the National Health Service, have been very slow to understand the realities of how food works and, in particular, its role in guarding against cancer. Hospitals still serve meals that are nutritionally useless and often harmful; more patients suffer from malnutrition than anyone admits. Yet food is medicine. The excuse is usually cut-backs or overwork but the real reason is ignorance.

Scientifically, a link between food and cancer has now been proved by eminent epidemiologists who have studied cancer trends worldwide. They say that constant unbalanced eating upsets body mechanics, creating devitalised toxic conditions in which tumours and other diseases thrive.

For instance, women living in countries with a low fat diet such as Japan appear to have less risk of breast cancer but, on the other hand, the huge amount of raw, pickled or spiced food eaten raises the incidence of stomach cancer. Bowel cancer is on the increase in high meat-eating countries, whereas cancer of any sort is rare amongst those who eat simple, unprocessed foods.

There is very little cancer in Africa and it is uncommon among pure living Mormons and Seventh Day Adventists in Utah, USA. The much studied 'Happy Valley' people of Hunza, northern India, where on average they live to be well over a hundred, is so far a UNESCO cancer-free zone. Hunzaputs lead quiet, unsophisticated lives on a diet of raw apricots and yoghurt. The soil is rich in the elements selenium and rubidium and there is no western medicine. Ironically, since the west discovered the Hunza Valley and its 'magic' apricots and Afghanistan seized an opportunity for a thriving export trade, we have introduced, in return, refined flour and sugar, since when recent reports say the legendary health is failing.

Hunza apricots now on sale in most good health food stores are delicious but are not necessarily from the valley.

In Iran, the high incidence of oesophagal cancer, one of the slowest and most painful types, hangs like a sword of Damocles over some 300,000 Turkoman tribesfolk. These people live in the desert and their basic food is bread. Some 300 miles away, in the damp, Caspian forests where the basic food is rice, the same people have only an average incidence of the disease. This phenomenon was first noted by the thirteenth century physician, Jurjani. Rather than seeking a specific cause for cancer, maybe we should be looking at the basic relationship between man and his environment ... the interplay between the external world and our responses to it.

Carcinogens can be found naturally in almost everything we eat but only rarely do they become a problem. If you are worried, any of the cancer centres, such as that at Bristol, will advise on sensible, no-fuss eating to suit you and your family.

When it comes to planning a sensible diet either for yourself or for a family, remember this is Britain — not Bolivia. Your local shop may waft with coriander and cumin these days, but we need to plan our eating around the place we live, the job we do, the ages of our dependents. The hair shirt approach to diet is not for all — there really is no harm in an impulsive take-away. Your children will not suffer from occasional fish fingers.

Good nutrition means a diet adequate in carbohydrate, protein, fat, vitamins, minerals and water, one that is balanced in its proportion of calories from carbohydrate (which should contribute more than 55 per cent of the daily calorie intake) from fat (less than 30 per cent) and from protein (approximately 15 per cent). So it is 'Yes' to ...

Natural foods There are up to 3,000 different additives used in Britain — half of them unnecessary. Their reactive effect one upon the other is, so far, unknown. By baking your own bread, with wholemeal flour, for instance, you can avoid 34 chemical ingredients used in some shop bought loaves. Additives are hugely controversial. The case against them is not proven. But the parents of any hyperactive child know the dramatic effect that removing colouring and flavour enhancers can have on the child's behaviour.

To meet today's demands for cheap international food distribution and mass marketing we are told food must be preserved and to give it sales appeal it is livened up with artificial flavouring and colour. The EEC has worked out a code which is designed to help shoppers decide for themselves which of the additives are genuinely necessary and which are there for the good of the manufacturer. It is then up to each individual to balance out the risk of eating tainted meat, for instance, against the risk of eating preservatives. Recently a campaign for 'real' meat has added its voice to the lobby.

For the conscientious, there is a book, *Additives – Your Complete Survival Guide*, which gives a breakdown of all artificial ingredients and their role. Many chain stores are introducing additive or sugar-free products in response to demand – but even these labels should be carefully read as manufacturers sometimes find loop-holes. When the packet of your supermarket apple pie says 'flour' it does not mention all the additives in the flour! In America, where manufacturers are 'guilty' until proved innocent, suspected toxins may not be added to food until proved safe. The reverse is true here where the use of an additive is permitted until it has been proved harmful.

Organic food in season. This not only tastes better, it really does you more good. Food grown artificially in nitrate-saturated soil is a potential health hazard and a mounting problem. Nitrates from fertilisers are converted into nitrites and subsequently into nitrosamines in the human body and these have been proved to be carcinogenic in tests on animals. Holland has brought in legislation to establish an upper limit for the safe use of nitrates in vegetable production – it was discovered that out of season hot-house lettuces, hearted-up under glass, were highly toxic. Switzerland has followed suit. In Britain we have done nothing.

Pulses are an excellent source of protein. Choose chick peas, lentils, mung beans, etc.

Sprouting grains and seeds contain a rich source of vitamin C and active enzymes: alfalfa, millet, buckwheat, cracked wheat, brown rice.

'Live' food and its aura

High voltage photographs can show up an 'aura' – a luminous

glow which appears to surround all living things. This has been claimed as the explanation of the 'halo' of mediaeval saints. Kirlian photography, named after the Russian engineer, S. Kirlian, who pioneered the method in 1939, reveals a vast difference between the energy of live food, such as an apple picked direct from the tree, and dead food which has been processed and stored. It is believed that the natural energies have then been replaced by chemical energies. Such luxuries as garden carrots may be out of reach of the inner city family but if that is the case – don't panic. Knowing the ideal, buy the freshest food you can.

Supplements

Most doctors recommend nutritional supplements today since these are not available in sufficient quantity in our over-processed food. This is why we have such a poor standard of nutrition, according to recent reports in *The Lancet*. Vitamins and minerals protect the immune system and should be taken on advice as part of a routine nutritional plan. In particular, we need:

Vitamin A or carotene Scientists believe there may be a link between carotene – the plant form of vitamin A – and a reduced incidence of cancer. Cancer cells produce a protein which inhibits the action of the immune system. Beta-carotene combines with this and neutralises its action. It is sensible in any case to include plenty of green, leafy vegetables and the yellow, orange vegetables such as carrots in your daily diet. But, for the body to absorb beta-carotene, capsules must be taken in emulsified form otherwise absorption is poor.

Vitamin B group The B vitamins have an essential role in promoting appetite and digestive tract functioning. They are very important in recovery from illness, and patients on chemotherapy or radiotherapy, for instance, need three times the usual amount of vitamin B. All B vitamins are water-soluble and cannot be stored for any length of time in the body so must be regularly replenished. The natural sources of Vitamin B are alfalfa sprouts and fresh green vegetables or brewer's yeast.

Vitamin C is one of the most unstable vitamins. It can be destroyed by exposing it to light and by heat. In its natural state, this, too, is a protection against cancer. It is best eaten in raw food but if cooked, vegetables or fruit should be left whole and cooked in a minimum amount of pre-boiled water. Choose oranges that have ripened naturally, if possible – most of those at the greengrocer's have been picked when unripe and injected with tartrazine to induce the orange colour. Their vitamin C content is, in fact, surprisingly low. Cauliflower, sprouts and spinach also contain vitamin C. Very large doses of vitamin C tablets can cause diarrhoea in cancer patients and it is best taken in a salt such as calcium ascorbate.

Vitamin D is sometimes called 'the bone vitamin' and is very important even after full growth has been achieved because bones are always changing. It is unique because the body synthesises its own vitamin D in the sunlight. Because the amount of ultra violet light from the sun varies according to season and locality, supplementary vitamin D is necessary, particularly in industrial societies and northern latitudes. It is found naturally in egg yolk, salmon, sardines, fish oils and yeast.

Vitamin E helps prevent the formation of free radicals, over-active atomic particles which damage the genetic structure of cells and can create cancerous conditions. Vegetable oils are a rich source of vitamin E which is also found in wheatgerm, eggs, fish, leafy vegetables and cereals.

Selenium There is an increasing amount of evidence from America that selenium is a cancer preventive. Norfolk is the only place in Britain where this element still occurs naturally in the soil. At the University of California, Dr Gerhard Schrauzer has found that supplementary selenium reduces cancer in animals treated with almost any carcinogen. Many people add selenium to their diet in tablet form; the maximum daily dose is 200 micrograms since large doses are toxic. Other sources are free range poultry, especially turkey, whole grains and seaweed.

Zinc, potassium and copper are needed by a number of

enzymes which help in protecting the immune system. They are all essential minerals sadly lacking in western diet, due largely to our destructive methods of farming. There are simple tests for mineral deficiency usually available from a good health centre. It may be wise to make up any short-fall with approved supplements, since there is no way of arriving at the necessary amount naturally.

Potassium occurs naturally in citrus fruits, watercress and bananas. Zinc is present in brewer's yeast, non-fat milk powder and mustard. Copper comes in kelp, onions and sea-food.

Optional Supplements

Ginseng helps to raise immunity and is a natural source of steroids which protect against stress and stress-related diseases. It should be taken only on advice and not continuously.

Evening primrose seed oil This supplies gamma linoleic acid, one of the essential fatty acids found only in plants. These develop into hormones which protect the genetic structure of cells and so help to shield the body against cancer.

Reduce or cut out:

Polysaturated animal fats Margarine, butter and other dairy products. The liver converts some fats to acids which are secreted as part of the bile into the gut. There, bacteria chemicals alter these bile acids into tumour growth-promoting material — so claim Drs Cohen and Reddy of the Naylor Dana Institute in America. Excess fats also inhibit the production of prostaglandin which has a protective and curative role.

Salt and allied additives such as monosodium glutamate (used as a flavour enhancer), sodium nitrite (added to meat and fish as a curing preservative), baking soda (a raising agent) and sodium phosphate (a wetting agent). Salt destroys potassium — much needed for the destruction of cancer cells. Instead, try seasoning with herbs, especially cumin and Selora (a commercially produced salt substitute). Sea salt is better than table salt, but it is best to avoid adding salt altogether.

Sugar Whether it is described as glucose, fructose, maltose or caramel, brown sugar is only a little better than white. Unblended honey in limited amounts is passable. There is no place for sugar in a cancer patient's diet. Many supermarkets now display jams made without added sugar for instance and, though their taste may at first strike harshly, persevere because the palate adapts and the full fruit taste is delicious.

Many canned or processed convenience foods are high in animal fats, salt and sugar, and should be eaten with discretion.

Meat The human intestine was not made to cope with meat, though many of us enjoy it. In moderation it probably does no harm and there are some people whose metabolism seems to need meat – even then white meat is probably preferable to beef and pork. Ask your butcher where he buys his meat and be sure he knows if it is free of hormone injections to aid growth since these are a feared cancer agent. On the whole, once a week – perhaps the Sunday roast – certainly does no harm, but much more than that is probably unwise.

Drinks Fresh, unsweetened juices (especially carrot) are better than over-coloured cordials. There are some natural chemicals present in tea and coffee which act as stimulants or depressants so these drinks are best kept to a sensible minimum. The caffeine in tea and, especially, in coffee interferes with enzyme production, and decaffeinated coffee is produced with a potentially carcinogenic component. Don't take a lot of liquid with meals – it tends to wash nutrients through before they are properly assimilated.

Alcohol Common sense dictates moderation at all times. Curiously, many people who develop cancer find that they 'go off' it altogether – the body seems to say 'enough'. But there is no need to become teetotal if social drinking is woven into your lifestyle. Just remember, neat spirits are to be treated warily. At 18 milligrams per cent blood level, alcohol begins to stimulate prostaglandin formation, so can be used as a pick-you-up or a night-cap occasionally!

The Vitamin Man

Dr Linus Pauling, professor of chemistry, winner of two Nobel prizes, has championed mankind in the battle against the dangers of twentieth century life for 40 years. He is 85 and confidently certain that we could, with a little reorganisation, all die healthy. We should consult doctors only when we are seriously ill. It is very important to realise that 'the decision to consult a doctor is a potentially risky one . . .'

His plan is extremely controversial – some say dangerous – but intriguing. He believes that this is the age of the vitamin – and that cancer, being a mega-disease, could be prevented by a mega-vitamin therapy.

Vitamin C, in particular, he sees as the Knight Errant, the essential guardian of the immune system. A vital role in the body's immune system is played by antibodies (see page 10). It has been found that when we increase our intake of vitamin C our bodies produce more of these antibody molecules.

'I have concluded that the optimum dose that should be taken regularly to preserve good health and provide protection against disease – including cancer – is between 260 and 4,000 milligrams a day – sometimes as much as 10,000.' Dr Pauling's plan for a long, healthy life includes daily massive doses of vitamins and minerals:

One 800 IU vitamin E capsule
One B complex tablet
One vitamin and mineral tablet
One 25,000 IU vitamin A capsule

Do *not* overdo the mineral intake – stick to prescribed doses or they can be dangerous.

Take your vitamin C (three level teaspoonsful) before breakfast and the rest in the evening dissolved in orange juice or water made fizzy with (he says) a little baking powder.

It is important to stick with the plan once started – don't let up for even a day. Cost, according to Dr Pauling, is no more than a can of fizzy drink a day . . . but prices do vary. Avoid vitamins with unnecessary rose hip powder added. On such a massive vitamin intake, Dr Pauling claims, there is less need to be obsessive about cutting down on animal fats.

For further information about Dr Pauling's plan, see his book *How to Live Longer and Feel Better*.

Laetrile

Laetrile/Amygdalin/'Vitamin' B17 is sometimes claimed to be to cancer what vitamin C was to scurvy. This is the conviction of those medical men worldwide who believe that the natural substance produced by apricot kernels, used wisely, is a powerful cytotoxic agent. But it is one of the most controversial anti-cancer substances available and is banned in the USA, ostensibly because it also contains an element of cyanide although organic cyanide, say its supporters, is harmless.

The term laetrile was introduced by Dr Ernest Krebs Sr of San Francisco in 1952. It is an amygdalin, which is a simple chemical compound consisting of two molecules of sugar, one molecule of benzaldehyde and one molecule of cyanide bound tightly together. Amygdalin was used by the Chinese 3,000 years ago in bitter almond essence, but it was first isolated in 1830 by French chemists Robiquet and Boutron Charland.

At the forefront of the laetrile movement was test pilot and businessman Andrew McNaughton, who set up the non-profitmaking, philanthropic McNaughton Foundation for the testing and development of laetrile. He says that primitive people who eat only organic, unfractionated or whole food regularly ingest 250–500 milligrams of cyanide each day. This natural cyanide, locked inside a sugar molecule, is normal to our metabolism and when eaten and taken into healthy cells is detoxified and released into the urine by the enzyme, rhodanese.

Cancer cells are deficient in rhodanese and are surrounded by a different enzyme, beta-glucosidase; this is secreted by the cell and, in turn, releases the bound cyanide from the amygdalin at the site of the malignancy and this cyanide destroys the cancer cells. Organic cyanide is, therefore, a highly selective substance 'which shoots the enemy only' – toxic to cancer cells, non-toxic to the rest.

The furore that has raged around laetrile has been dramatic for such a simple substance. There have been charges of dishonesty and corruption on both sides although there is no commercial profit to be made by its extraction. This is easily and inexpensively done and, therefore, is of no interest to drug companies. It could even be considered a threat. The medical establishment argue that it is a hoax, dangerous and a hazard to patients who might be side-tracked from orthodox treatment by its use.

Advocates of laetrile do not claim it is a cure – more a cancer prevention treatment, and that all too often patients resort to it too late, when all else has failed. It has been found to be more effective in some cancers than others. Doctors in Israel, for instance, found that Hodgkin's disease responded, but that it had little value in leukaemia. Interestingly, some of the best results have been with lung cancer.

Amygdalin therapy is only useful if applied in conjunction with a completely vegetarian diet and a metabolic approach to food – in other words, it is a part of a holistic treatment. It is given orally or by injection and its effects range from diminished pain, nausea control and increased appetite, through to tumour shrinkage, depending on dosage, quality of support, extent of the tumour and damage already done from radiation, chemotherapy or surgery.

Laetrile occurs naturally in many plants and so can be taken as a cancer preventive simply by including certain foods on the daily menu. These include chick peas, watercress, alfalfa, bean sprouts, nuts, mung beans, blackberries, gooseberries, raspberries, the stones and seeds of the apple, apricot, cherry, nectarine, plum and pear. It can be bought in health stores in tablet form but should not be taken without the advice of a qualified practitioner. For further information, contact Leon Chaitow (sae, please) c/o Thorsons Publishers, see Useful Addresses.

'The Uneasy Passions of the Mind'

Stress, tension and trauma are fashionable words for an age old problem. The link between stress and the onset of cancer was pondered by Galen in 38 AD and 1,700 years later by J. Burrows. In 1783 Burrows wrote 'Cancer is caused by the uneasy passions of the mind.' Today, we would not say that it is 'caused' by stress, rather that the conditions for its beginning are set up.

Stress is not something that happens from outside. In his book *The Gate of Healing*, Dr Ian Pearce says 'Life is full of challenges. These do not of themselves constitute stress. Stress is what we create in ourselves by the way in which we meet the challenge.' There can be as much stress in an apparently tranquil nunnery as in the office of an advertising company.

On the other hand, the tragedy of war itself, for instance, does not necessarily cause stress. Quite the opposite – it 'stiffens the sinews' – gets us going. We are often at our best in a national crisis. Cancer incidence dropped dramatically during the Second World War and rose again when the challenge of wartime conditions was lifted.

One of the world's most respected authorities on the psychology of cancer is Lawrence Le Shan. In a massive programme of research carried out over 17 years in the United States, he became sure there is a cancer-prone personality. He has devoted much of his life to educating such people to make adjustments in their attitudes so that they can cope with situations that might otherwise become dangerous.

The events which seem to cause the greatest threat of cancer are:

- Death of spouse
- Divorce
- Sexual problems within marriage
- The bachelor state
- Job loss

All these are concerned with a long-term sense of isolation and rejection, or the loss or absence of a central relationship. (Very often, if this occurs within a marriage, children fill the gap.) This, says Le Shan, is the characteristic of cancer – it is 'foiled creative fire'.

> Nobody knows what the cause is
> Though some pretend they do
> It's like some hidden assassin
> Waiting to strike at you
> Childless women get it
> And men when they retire
> It's as if there had to be some outlet
> For their foiled creative fire.
>
> *W. H. Auden*

Kate's experience seems a hard way to learn.

Is it possible to change the emotional programme we are all born with? Can we steer a course that helps us feel more at peace without needing to contract cancer?

Certainly, it is now known that mind *can* rule over matter.

Kate's Story – A Cold Life

Kate had been a recording and rehearsal studio manager – a bachelor girl living alone. At the age of 54 she was in St Joseph's Hospice, in London, with advanced carcinoma of the jaw. She had read no books on cancer or psychology – she had never heard of Lawrence Le Shan. Her story was exactly as he described.

'I was a very outgoing person and lived a very open life. I'd lived with various guys, I loved sailing and had a pretty good time. Yet it was a cold life. I was always cold inside. Looking back now, I can see what was missing was a real close relationship, a family, love.

'I developed agoraphobia – I suppose I needed attention. That kept me away from my dentist – and so I allowed what I thought was an abscess to get out of hand. It wasn't an abscess, of course.

'Here in St Joseph's, I have felt the warm glow of friendship for the first time. Somehow I have become a real person – I'm not role playing any more. I'm not competing with the outside world. Some people turn to God – not me. I just feel I am living through a real life experience – death is real, what is happening to us is real, and somehow my having cancer has not been a totally negative experience at all. It has contributed to my life. I don't really know why this is – I am literally feeling my way through the experience like reading Braille, and now the world is warm and I have such deep feelings for the first time.'

That we can, with guidance, learn consciously to change our pulse rate, heartbeat and temperature. This is what Biofeedback is all about (see page 47). Positive and negative thoughts induce the production of different sets of chemicals by the brain. Lawrence Le Shan says

... since all these secretions are directly involved in the maintenance of health and in overcoming disease, one thing appears likely: under circumstances of depression, fear, panic, exasperation and frustration, the healing resources of the brain are not fully engaged.

I believe potentially vulnerable individuals can create a degree of psychological immunity that will increase their chances of resisting disease. Amongst those stricken, the people most capable of recovery are men and women who can discover a new well spring of hope, whatever their past disappointments, and move on to a fresh sense of themselves, a true recognition of their needs and of their worth as human beings.

Not all human illnesses, of course, are treatable through self-control techniques, but medical intervention works much better when the resources of the patient are fully engaged. The physician knows that his medications can be much more effective when patients have the will to live.

The pattern forms at birth. Parents can hand on to their offspring not only genetically based strengths and weaknesses but they do to a large extent direct their emotional development. It is possible to create a non-cancerous environment for childhood. *A child needs constant reassurance of love — by cuddling, touching. He must be taught pride in himself, learn to play and to create. The much criticised ability to 'express himself' is a vital outlet.*

So often, cancer patients have been lonely, isolated and instilled with a feeling of self-dislike and even guilt about inadequacy — 'If I'm good, Mummy will love me.' They have failed to 'bond' with either parent, feel jealous of brothers or sisters or that there is 'something wrong' with themselves. They begin to transform who they are, to what they think they are expected to be. That is where it all goes wrong. It is vital, too, to be aware just as much of what we *feel* as what we do. Everyone has strongly personal individual characteristics which are unlike anyone else's. It is essential to understand what these are and to build upon them — to sing your own tune.

To live for someone else is not enough. When that person is no longer there, or there is any catastrophe to overcome, the support collapses. Each one of us must learn first to believe in ourselves, to become 'the master of my fate, the captain of my soul'.

Sometimes, this may mean acting like a lobster. The lobster has a thick outside shell and the only way he can grow is to shed the shell that protects him. This can be a painful process. It means asking questions not like 'What do I want to do with my life?' but 'What do I feel about my life right now?'

Finding the answer to such questions can be tough. Everyone needs a friend, a counsellor, someone to confide in. Even men, whose emotions from birth are so often 'in armour clad', need an outlet. Ignore that at your peril. Some find support in an individual – maybe a priest or a lover. Others can be greatly strengthened by joining a religious group whose common interest is a search for peace of mind. Others again find help in the pursuit of physical and mental health, along the routes of nutrition, exercise, sport and spiritual exploration.

Beware the pill bottle. It is only too easy to become addicted not only to heroin or other hard drugs but to tranquillisers and pep pills. The withdrawal symptoms from these can be as painful as the 'cold turkey' treatment undergone by hard drug addicts.

If you are in need of help, try instead your local counselling service (there are now hundreds of trained men and women available nationwide at a minimal cost tailored to your pocket), or the nearest branch of the National Marriage Guidance Council, which helps families too. They are good on the nitty gritty stress of everyday life – for deeper, more long term emotional problems, you may need a specialist.

Biofeedback

Biofeedback is a means of increasing awareness of mental states by understanding the body's responses with the help of a simple monitoring machine. In its simplest form, for instance, a patient can learn to raise or lower his own temperature. There are many kinds of Biofeedback machine used to measure electrical resistance of the skin, brain wave patterns and muscle tension. Once the technique is taught, a patient can control his own blood pressure and minimise illnesses where tension is a problem.

Because Biofeedback is a relaxation technique, it is most effective in easing the kind of stress that leads to illnesses such as cancer, rather than as a cure. Its place is preventive and it is increasingly accepted as such, even by orthodox practitioners.

Not Tonight, Josephine?

Sexuality is a fundamental pivot of life, alongside eating and breathing. You may choose to deflect that force into a different area but you should never underestimate its role in preserving wellness. The relationship between love, the emotion, and sex, the energy, is complex, yet an understanding of this part of your personality could be an important precaution in caring for your health.

Richard Wells, at the Royal College of Nursing, is one of the few people in Britain specialising in the study of cancer and sexuality. He believes 'We do not give nearly enough credence to what the body tells us. Very often I find that loss of libido predates a diagnosis of cancer – carcinogens have a flattening effect on the personality. So never allow your sex worries to go unaided at any age.'

Of course, different people have different appetites. Some people live apparently happy, celibate lives, but a change in the norm, or a build-up of tension or anxiety should never be ignored. When 'the urge' goes, or things between you and a partner have physically 'gone off the boil' and if you are distressed about it, don't keep the distress to yourself. GPs should always ask patients about their personal relationships rather than hand out tranquillisers but all too often they will assume a female patient is neurotic. Very few men are prepared to discuss such things at all. If that is the case, try a Marriage Guidance Counsellor.

Enquiries can be sent to the Psychosexual Unit at the Royal Maudsley Hospital, London. Or private patients can go to the Institute for Sex Education Research (see Useful Addresses).

Bittersweet Pill

The pill is a problem. There is a great deal of contradictory evidence about its links with cervical and breast cancer. In 1984, scare stories in the Press were provoked by an article in *The Lancet* and were then categorically denied by other medical journals and a number of family planning organisations. More recently, the *Journal of Alternative Medicine* said 'There is now a well-established link between the use of the contraceptive pill and subsequent deficiency of vitamin B6'. As many cervical cancer patients also reveal a B6 deficiency, the conclusion is: the pill equals B6 deficiency equals cancer.

The risks clearly have to be set in the context of the needs of the individual and of the community in which she lives. In an

African village the chance of death from cancer is probably less than from starvation due to over-population. We also have to take on board the complex web of moral and religious attitudes and the, so far, unknown genetic effects. In today's western society, the danger of unwanted pregnancy is perhaps more of an issue. So what is a girl to do?

The Family Planning Association will advise individual cases, for each set of circumstances may require a different approach. Contact them locally, or at their London headquarters (see Useful Addresses). The Brook Advisory Centre, too, is a well-respected source of advice and information on all aspects of sex and contraception, especially for the young unmarried (see Useful Addresses).

Body Maintenance

There is nothing neurotic about regular maintenance of machinery – the body included. The aim of any early warning system for cancer is to detect the disease at a stage in its natural development when it is containable. In the case of breast and cervical tests, the benefits are on the whole well-established – though not undisputed. There are those who say that pre-cancerous conditions and even lumps found by tests might well have gone away of their own accord anyway and that such discovery can only create needless worry.

Cervical Smears

There is as yet no nationally or even regionally organised screening programme in Britain although it was announced last year that a national computerised system would shortly be set up. In this, we have lagged behind many other countries. This is probably why there has been some controversy over the value of the examination. Even so, screening for cervical cancer is the longest established screening process in Britain and is unique because it picks up a pre-cancerous condition. This does not mean that malignancy is always present, only that, in one third of positive cases, it could be, if neglected. The danger age is after 35, and this is why GPs are not encouraged (indeed, not paid yet) to do smears for younger women. But the demand is growing for tests to be available for all sexually active women, and the BMA now recommends that, ideally, any woman between the age of 20 and 60 should be tested at three yearly intervals.

The good news is that only one in 500 to 700 cases is positive . . . which, of course, throws into question the cost effectiveness of the entire scheme. Leon Chaitow (*An End to Cancer*) argues that the money might be better spent on educating adolescents in hygiene.

What happens You go along to your doctor who may do a test in the surgery. The test is done painlessly by taking cells from the cervix with a spatula. If there is a delay, find out where else you can go. Alternative testing centres are the free mobile clinics run by the Women's National Cancer Control Campaign (which are available on request to local authorities and businesses and tour the country). Testing is also available at FPA clinics, Well Woman clinics and cytology centres. Private health insurance companies such as BUPA run their own scheme and liaise with many commercial companies who encourage employees to keep a check on their health.

The sample cells are then sent to laboratories for analysis and this is where problems usually begin. There is often a disconcerting wait for results and there are occasions when the results are inaccurate or even wrong. This can cause tremendous distress. These delays – sometimes up to 6 months – are due to a shortage of laboratory staff; screeners are usually part time because it is not possible to do close microscope work for long periods. Some private labs do not have a consultant pathologist and, occasionally, samples are even sent away to Sweden for analysis. No wonder there is a hold-up. There is also concern that some borderline cases may be treated unnecessarily. If you don't receive a reply at all, do not assume all is well. Go back . . . again and again. Results can be swallowed up in the system and dangerous delays result.

If the initial tests reveal some abnormality, then further tests will be necessary. The grading of the disease is recorded as CIN (Cervical Intraepithelial Neoplasia) and the degree of problem measured from CIN 1 and 2, which is mild to moderate dyskaryosis, to CIN 3, which is malignant carcinoma in situ. In any of these cases, examination with a colposcope is the best course. This is a microscope which can see the entire cervix and locate exactly the extent of the trouble. Sadly, colposcopes are expensive and available in far fewer NHS hospitals than in the private sector. If there is no colposcope in the area, a cone biopsy may be done to remove a ring of the cervix and this procedure is available in all NHS hospitals. Women with CIN 1 or 2 may find that on a second check 3 months later the problem has reverted of its own accord, but in these cases a further test after 3 months is a sensible precaution.

Breast Checks

The do-it-yourself breast check should be a once a month routine. (See overleaf for instructions on how to do this.) The biggest risk is that it can turn women into hypochondriacs — especially as many have naturally 'granular' or lumpy breasts and find the difference between normality and irregularity hard to detect. It is a good idea to ask your doctor to do a check whenever you are in his surgery.

A breast lump should be seen by a hospital immediately. It is not for the GP to decide that it is safe to leave. It should be considered guilty until proven innocent. Eighty per cent of all lumps are not cancerous.

Mammography Sometimes patients at special risk will be referred for a mammography. This is an X-ray technique designed to detect lumps too small to be felt manually. There are not many such units in Britain and there is often a delay for National Health patients. Privately this screening facility costs around £50.

This, too, is a controversial method of diagnosis because it involves a very high dosage of radiation, which believers in a gentler approach would say is likely, in fact, to stimulate the cancer. It is also not very reliable. If you are in doubt, it may be wise to discuss your personal story with a specialist trained in orthodox and complementary medicine.

Help from: WNCCC (Women's National Cancer Control Campaign); Family Planning Association (for both, see Useful Addresses).

Dental Visits

It is the dentist, more often than not, who spots oral cancer. It is fortunately rare, tending to appear as a white patch or ulcer

Breast examination

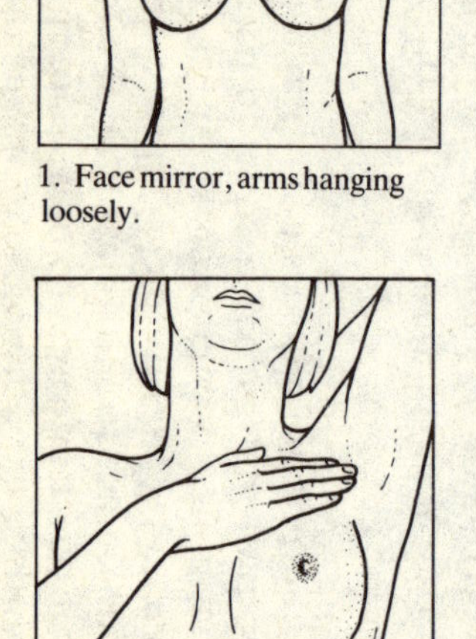

1. Face mirror, arms hanging loosely.

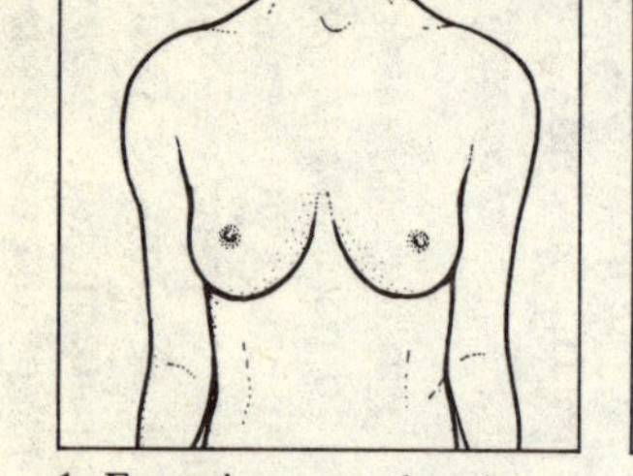

2. Raise arms. Turn from side to side.

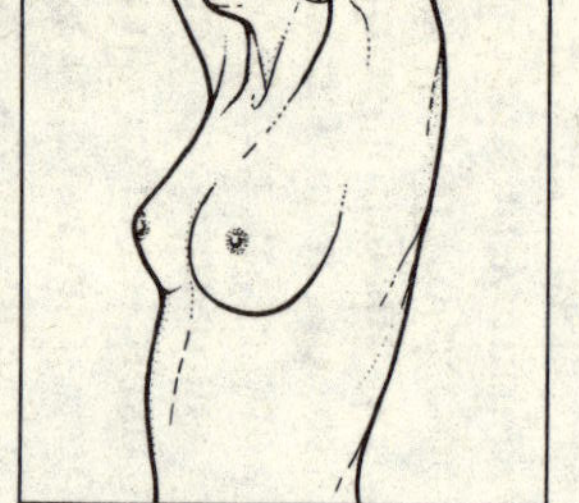

3. Squeeze nipples. Check for unusual discharge.

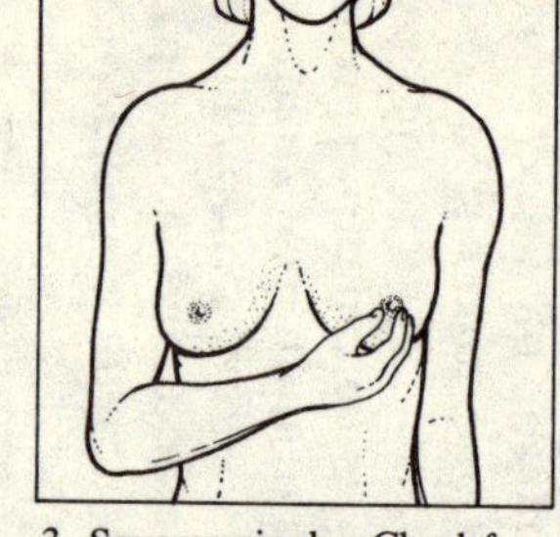

4. Lie down. Head on pillow. Fold towel under left shoulder, then right, one hand under head. Examine each breast, fingers together and flat.

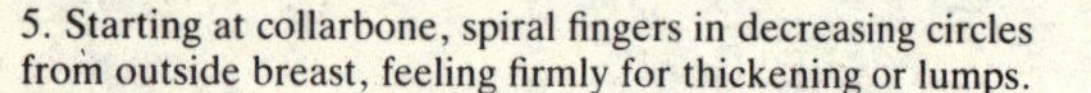

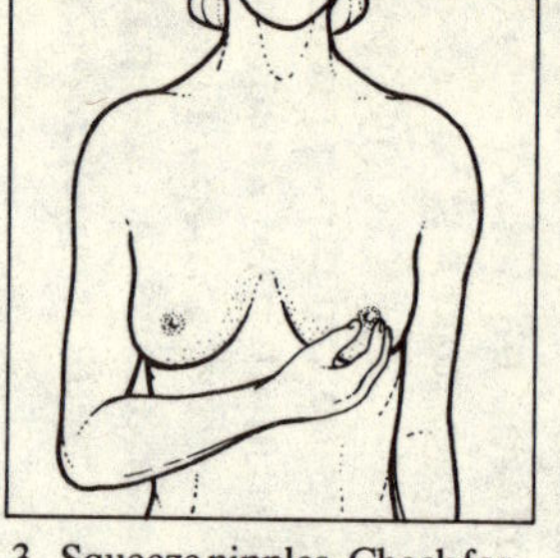

5. Starting at collarbone, spiral fingers in decreasing circles from outside breast, feeling firmly for thickening or lumps. The half-moon of firm tissue beneath breasts is normal.

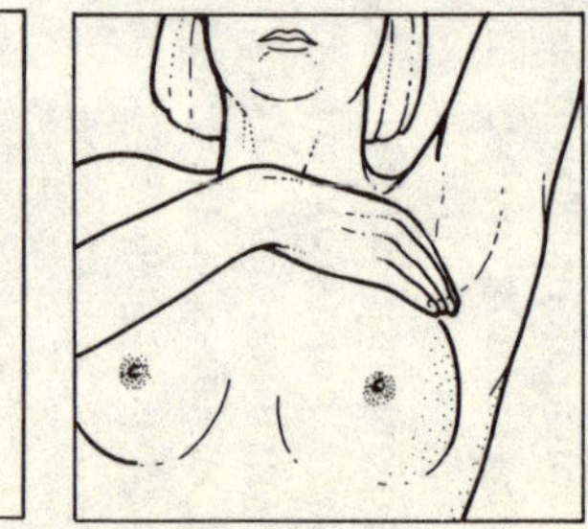

6. Examine armpit in same way, from the hollow downwards.

which only he will see. Oral cancer is often associated with non-European habits such as tobacco-chewing, but also with excessive drinking, smoking and injury. But a dental check is common sense anyway to avoid dentures and pain.

The Exercise Man

'The good life is bad for you', says Dr Jan de Winter, former senior consultant at the Royal Sussex County Hospital and pioneer of the world's first cancer whole body scanner, as well as founder of the Brighton Cancer Prevention Foundation. He sees life as a 'three-legged stool': nutrition, exercise and peace of mind – each indispensable. 'If you haven't the time to exercise, you should rearrange your life.' Exercise, he says, produces endorphines, which have a morphia-like calming effect on the body. It also increases the 'stroke volume' – the amount of blood the heart pushes out, increasing oxygen supply to the body. By far the best exercise, he says, is swimming – followed by cycling or running, soft jogging, or even a fast walk.

'We are a precious mechanism,' he says, 'and should be treated with care. I believe in the maintenance of health – whereas in medical schools we are taught to control disease, nothing is taught about nutrition or preventive medicine. We have been a closed shop with a closed mind – but in 20 years things will be better. But I do not believe in forcing anything on anyone, and if people don't want to be helped then you can't help. There are so many people who do desperately need counsel it is not for me to try and convert those who don't care.'

Help from: Dr Jan de Winter, The Brighton Cancer Prevention Foundation (see Useful Addresses).

High Risk Jobs?

You can't choose your job for its cancer rating. That kind of neurosis would bring industry and commerce to its knees. Clearly, some work entails higher risk than others, but if you come from a family of miners or long line of sugar refiners you are more likely to accept those risks . . . especially as many of the potentially life-threatening substances take years to be proved guilty. There was 30 years' research before the link between workers producing zinc chromate pigments and lung cancer was confirmed.

The discovery or confirmation of long standing risks has been helped by improved epidemiological research which, in theory, should make prevention easy because manufacturers should be able to remove the offending substance. In practice, because truth is so hard to establish, manufacturers sometimes have their eye on cash rather than cancer.

The earliest and best-known example of industrial cancer is that of the climbing boys – the apprentice sweeps who scaled eighteenth-century chimneys. These children were discovered to suffer frequently from cancer of the scrotum by a surgeon at St Bartholomew's Hospital, named Percivall Pott. This, he found, was caused by the rubbing of carcinogenic soot-covered hands on the naked body. Climbing boys were abolished – and cancer of the scrotum virtually disappeared.

Of course, any job can take its health toll. Both writer's cramp and farmer's lung are officially DHSS prescribed industrial diseases!

Because there is no money for research there is no certain proof of many industrial carcinogens. Current worry amongst ecologists is PVC. Could there be a link between plastic greenhouses and an increased incidence of brain tumours in horticulturalists? Who knows the effects of plasticised wall-papers and paints in children's bedrooms? How did we live without cling film? There are those who fear we may not live with it and that the hygienic supermarket wrap transfers carcinogens to our food. Best remove it as soon as possible. Some of the proven defaulters are:

- Asbestos – which triggers mesothelioma (cancer of the chest)
- Benzene in rubber manufacture – provokes leukaemia and lymphoma
- Ionising radiation arising from the nuclear industry
- Woodworkers' materials and occupational environment – woodworkers sometimes suffer from nasal cancer

Should you contract cancer and believe it to have arisen

through your job, you should go to your nearest Citizens' Advice Bureau for help. There *is* a mechanism for making a claim through the DHSS against your employer or for a widow to claim for her husband's death, whether or not you have paid National Insurance contributions, but the process is slow and satisfying the adjudicating authorities is not always easy. As well as the leaflets listed below there is also a DHSS book outlining new disease reporting regulations, which puts the onus on the employer.

Help from: DHSS leaflets NI 2 and NI 196 on *Prescribed Industrial Diseases*, obtainable from HM Stationery Office, High Holborn, London WC2, or local DHSS.

Insurance

Being rejected by a life insurance company is like having a cheque bounced, failing a driving test or being found guilty in court. It is a vote of 'no confidence' and best avoided. Obviously, the time to protect your life against illness is *now* . . . before you become what brokers poetically call 'an impaired life'.

But if, like making a will, getting life insurance is on the list of jobs yet to be done, it is not too late to get cover even after a diagnosis of cancer.

Look through the Yellow Pages under Life, for a broker who specialises in this. He should help you locate a company who will welcome 'impaired life' policies. You can insure with them whether or not you are ill, as an extra safeguard. There is a considerable difference in attitudes between one company and another. Some are very conservative and won't handle clients with a history of cancer but there are reliable and competitive firms happy to do so. Much will depend on the type of tumour and spread. With cases of 'carcinoma in situ', such as cervical cancer, it is sometimes possible to be covered soon after treatment. With others, cover is given a varying number of years after completion of treatment, often with an additional premium payable for a limited period.

If you have already taken out a policy with one of the private health insurance companies – such as BUPA or PPP – and cancer is diagnosed, you are covered for any treatment recommended by your consultant up to the cut-off period of 180 days in hospital. This includes chemotherapy, surgery and radiotherapy, as well as homoeopathy, acupuncture and any complementary treatment authorised by a qualified specialist. They do not look happily on an applicant who already has cancer.

Since costs and rules are frequently being revised, for up to date information contact BUPA and PPP (see Useful Addresses).

Fluoride – Help or Hazard?

Because water is literally on tap, we take it for granted. But water is the source of a great many ills – some of them man-induced through chemical additives. Fluoride is one of these.

The great lobby guns for and against fluoride face each other across very stormy waters. The experts on either side are formidable; the evidence totally contradictory; the householder a pawn in between. The House of Commons debate on the Fluoride Bill in 1985 kept MPs up all night firing on all cylinders. The Bill empowered local authorities to add fluoride to the local water supply at the rate of one milligram per litre. The addition of fluoride is said to prevent dental decay but if a resident feels that the price being paid is *cancer* on tap he has no choice but to move or use only bottled water.

Fluorides occur naturally in water in varying proportions. They are toxic. The fluoride now being added to drinking water by some local authorities is an industrial waste product and is believed by many people to be carcinogenic.

The Argument Against
'Fluoride causes more human cancer deaths and it causes it faster than any other chemical,' says Dean Burk, Chief Chemist Emeritus, National Cancer Institute of America.

The 1920s and 1930s saw an astronomical growth of the aluminium and phosphate fertiliser industries. This gave rise to an unexpected pollution problem: fluoride. Fluoride pollution of the air damaged wildlife, crops and livestock. There were lawsuits which forced companies to instal pollution control devices to trap fluoride waste products but then came the crunch. What to do with this excess? Fluoride is not biodegradable. It was America which solved the problem: put it in drinking water 'on the pretext that it was good for teeth'. In his book, *The Ageing Factor*, John Yiamouyiannis, one of the world's leading fluoride authorities, fiercely attacks the American health establishment. He claims fluoride damages the body's repair and rejuvenation processes, that it attacks the immune system and that there is no safe level.

DNA is inhibited by fluoride, he says. If damage occurs to a cell which gives rise to a sperm or egg cell, that weakness or damage is passed on to the offspring. That means that, whilst cancer itself is not hereditary, the genetic weakness that makes a man or woman susceptible may be passed from generation to generation.

In Britain, according to the National Pure Water Association, dental decay is not caused by lack of fluoride. The Department of Health and Social Security agrees that the problem is over-indulgence in sticky sweets, ice cream, lollies and sweetened drinks . . . there has never been any positive proof of the value of fluoride.

In Sweden, Denmark, Norway and the Netherlands, fluoridation is illegal. It has never been accepted as safe in France or Italy and pilot schemes in Germany, Belgium and Switzerland have been stopped. In regions of these countries and in the USA cancer rates have risen when fluoride is added.

The anti-fluoride lobby points out that, just as no surgeon has the right to operate on a patient against his will, no one would dare suggest force-feeding with fluoride tablets. Summing up, they say 'Fluoridation brings in surreptitiously what no one would have dared bring in by the front door.'

The Argument For
Says BUPA in its *Manual of Fitness and Wellbeing*, 'this is the most effective way of supplying people with fluorine salts and no harm has ever been demonstrated.'

Professors Richard Doll and Peto also dismiss the anti-fluoride lobby in their book *The Causes of Cancer*. Fluoride, they say, occurs in its natural form in concentrations of up to 5.8 milligrams per litre. That is four times the dose allowed by the Act.

The BMA, the British Dental Association, the Royal College of Surgeons, the Royal College of General Practitioners and the Royal Commission on the National Health Service have all carried out studies and opted in favour of fluoride. The Royal Commission went even further: 'We are certain that it is entirely wrong to deprive the most vulnerable section of the population of such an important health measure for the sake of the views of a small minority of adults.'

To that Dr Yiamouyiannis would reply, referring to the state of play in the United States: 'To save their reputation, the promotors of fluoridation have intimidated, slandered, lied, destroyed and even corrupted the legislative, judicial and administrative bodies of our government.'

But that's America. It couldn't happen here . . . ? Or could it?

Help from: Nick Brugge, Secretary: National Pure Water Association; Mrs Maureen Lange, Administrator: The British Fluoridation Society (for both see Useful Addresses).

The Warning Signs

The cancer vigilante becomes a bore. Yet, once malignancy is diagnosed, it is human nature to look back and wonder where it all went wrong and regret those unheeded early warnings.

You know if you smoke. In your heart, you know if your marriage and/or sex life is sound, if your job is fulfilling, if you are abusing your body. If in doubt and you detect additional niggling symptoms there's no need to be afraid of talking to your doctor. The appearance of any one of these signs does *not* automatically mean cancer and may have some innocent explanation but, unless you are a fatalist, neither should they be neglected:

- Change in bowel or bladder habits
- A sore that doesn't heal
- Unusual bleeding or discharge
- Thickening or lumps
- Indigestion or difficulty in swallowing
- Obvious change in colour, size or bleeding of a mole or wart
- Nagging cough or hoarseness

Add to this the much vaguer, and possibly even earlier, changes that can precede cancer:

- Weight change, either loss or gain
- Personality change – irritability and dramatic changes of mood
- Dietary fads and unexpected change of taste
- Unpleasant bodily smells
- Loss of sex drive

Family or friends are often aware of these shifting patterns first. Is it ethical to take such suspicions to the doctor secretly, behind the patient's back? Most doctors will not act until the patient presents himself but will be glad to be put on the alert.

When you go to the doctor with one or more of these symptoms, you are probably already anxious. The decision to admit there could be something wrong feels like sitting at the top of a slippery slope. Of course the fears may be groundless. Of course there are a thousand and one more likely explanations than the one lurking at the back of the mind. If you are suspicious that it's cancer you should tell him – it will put him on his mettle and ensure a thorough, mind-settling examination. Frankness will also make your relationship easier.

The consultation should include: a check on your family health history, questions about your general well-being, your job, your family life, shocks or traumas; a physical examination, especially of the armpits, chest, groin and all body cavities, blood and urine and, for women, a cervical smear.

Should he dismiss your fears and say it is 'all in the mind' you can accept his word, or tell him you are still uneasy and take your troubles to the nearest Natural Health Centre that offers full medical checks by qualified staff.

You have the right to change your GP by letter if you can't face the personal interview, but practicalities dictate a choice within sensible visiting distance of your home. Your local Family Practitioners' Committee holds a list of all GPs under contract to them and the Medical Directory available in your local library lists doctors and their specialities. A useful book is *The Patient's Guide to the National Health* with a foreword by Katharine Whitehorn.

Help from: Your local Family Practitioner Committee and Community Health Council, both listed in your local telephone directory; *Medical Directory*, in the reference section of most public libraries.

4
Testing Time

The word 'tests' has a cold ring about it. Already you are entering a new world, one in which you may be very unsure of your ground. Even at this stage, be brave – think positive. This is the time to practise making friends with the medical team around you; if you never see them again, fine, but if you find yourself returning to the hospital for treatment later, you will have eased the path ahead.

Being friendly to doctors does not mean handing your fate to them on a plate. Decide before you set foot in the hospital what kind of patient you want to be. How much do you want to know? What do you want them to tell you? Patients should be seen *and* heard, but conversation is better than confrontation. It is your body – your life. You do have a right to question and to reject.

Most tests are quite safe, but in many there are varying degrees of discomfort. You will need to know:

- Why is the test necessary?
- How will it be done?
- What will I need to do?
- How painful is it?
- What are the side effects?
- How long does it take?
- Do I stay in hospital?
- Can I go home on my own afterwards?

Waiting for the results may leave you in suspense for days – or, sometimes, weeks. When they come, it is usually your own doctor who will tell you what they say (see chapter 5). If you have any reason for concern about accuracy you *can* ask for a second test in a different hospital – especially if you are attending a local general and would feel safer with a specialist centre. Tests are mostly accurate but mistakes *are* made. It is sometimes difficult to locate a hidden tumour and cancer can lurk undetected. On the other hand, if the tests are positive — even experts can be wrong. It's often a question of gut feelings. If you have obvious undisputed symptoms that are backed up by the result, it is probably correct. But if you have a borderline 'funny feeling', or the symptoms are less certain, then you may be wise to have a double check.

Already you have choices to make. Some of the alternative diagnostic methods are very sensitive. Many GPs will raise an eyebrow if this is your decision. All good holistic practitioners expect to work in tandem with the local doctor and some may suggest hospital tests as well. Going to a holistic doctor does not prevent you from turning to a hospital for treatment later, or vice versa. With many complementary methods, diagnosis and treatment are very closely linked. It is difficult to separate them since practitioners mostly see their main influence as preventive before curative, so acupuncture, reflexology and geopathic stress are included at this stage of the journey, though each has a role in the treatment of cancer too.

At the Hospital

Blood Tests

Blood testing is a means of identifying deficiencies. The samples are sent to the Haematology Department and to Chemical Pathology to measure enzymes. One of the warning signs the lab technicians will look for is the rate at which the red cells sink to the bottom of the test tube. They call this the ESR (erythrocyte sedimentation rate). These tests are painless, unless you are needle phobic. They are helpful in spotting leukaemia and sometimes bone marrow or liver problems.

Cytology

This is the branch of medicine dealing with the formation, structure and function of cells. The doctors will be investigating cells taken either from the urine or sputum, or from smears of the nose, mouth, lungs or cervix — the PAP test — or washings from the stomach. There are structural differences between cancer cells and others which can be spotted under a microscope, but generally speaking if there is something 'odd', doctors like to do a biopsy, too, for confirmation.

Biopsy
This is probably the test known best to the layman but it is also that which rings most alarm bells. The purpose of a biopsy is to prove that any abnormal mass or tumour is benign. Sometimes it is performed under local anaesthetic – tissue is taken from the suspect area for analysis, sometimes during one of the other tests such as the endoscopy. Sometimes exploratory minor surgery is necessary. The samples are studied by the pathologist.

A frozen section is the method of preparing tissue for immediate examination while the patient is still under anaesthetic. A permanent section subjects the tissue to a much more accurate examination and takes considerably longer to prepare.

At this stage a woman, in particular, needs her wits about her. She may be asked to sign a form agreeing to a radical mastectomy then and there if a breast lump proves malignant. Keep cool. This is *not necessary*. Some doctors still take the 'get it over and done with' line, and believe they save a woman from prolonged anxiety.

Before having a breast biopsy, any woman should be sure of her own feelings. She should not be hustled. There is nothing wrong in playing for time. A week's delay will not be a matter of life and death and will allow the chance of family discussion about the full implications of the verdict. She may even wish to refuse a mastectomy altogether and opt for alternative forms of treatment. She may feel an operation is the most reliable route to take. Not a decision to make in the frightening lead-up to a biopsy, and certainly not one to make until she has the result. Not until that 'guilty m'lud' verdict arrives can she be sure how she will react.

Occasionally, a suspicious lump – especially external tumours of the skin – may be removed complete for examination during a biopsy. It is wise to resist the needle biopsy of solid tissue which punctures the body's protective wall and leaves a passage along which malignant cells can escape. It is only justified for the removal of fluid.

Any patient has the right to query the biopsy result and ask for a second opinion – although since the emergence of oncology as a specialist subject doctors tend to consult more with each other before giving the thumbs down.

Lymph node biopsy The neck lumps you can feel when a child has tonsillitis are lymph nodes. Similar glands are scattered throughout the body and they mark the possible route of cancer spread. A lymph node biopsy may be done under either general or local anaesthetic according to its siting and is a simple out-patient job. Results can take several days.

Bone marrow biopsy Bone marrow is the blood-forming element within the bone, and is sucked out by a small needle under local anaesthetic. It is minimally painful – depending on the quality of the anaesthetic, but there is usually some bruising afterwards. If you are especially sensitive to pain, ask for additional tranquillisers; it is all over in a moment but there is no need to suffer. The results should be obtainable within a few hours.

Liver biopsy The test itself takes only half an hour under local anaesthetic, but the patient may be asked to stay overnight since very occasionally there are complications – maybe slight internal bleeding or bile leakage. Most patients may go home the same day but may be glad of a friend's company in case they feel a little queasy.

Pleural biopsy If fluid collects in the pleural cavity between the lung and chest wall, a biopsy of the chest wall will determine the reason. This is also a local anaesthetic job and the degree of discomfort as the lining is removed will, again, depend on the amount of anaesthetic. Any chesty pain should be reported immediately to the doctor. A chest X-ray should be performed after the test to ensure there has been no air leak from the lung itself. The test lasts only half an hour.

Skin biopsy Small areas of abnormal skin can be removed in a painless punch process lasting a few seconds. Larger areas may mean the removal of skin under local anaesthetic and stitching of the resultant small wound. Occasionally, a nasty mole or suspect skin growth may be removed altogether under full anaesthetic, but the reasons for taking this action should be fully discussed first with the patient, especially if there is any question of skin grafting.

X-Rays

There is so much to take on trust in the X-ray procedure. In a simple X-ray there is nothing to see, nothing to feel — and, therefore, in most of us, a niggly fear. This is not made easier by the fact that so many X-ray departments are tucked away in the bowels of the hospital or at the back of the oldest part of the building.

X-rays are one of the most useful diagnostic tools and are used to detect many kinds of cancer. Abnormal growth or accumulated tissue shows up darker than normal organs. They are not entirely without risk of radiation, itself stimulating cancer, but this has to be offset against the benefit.

You can ask the radiologist what dose you will be given — as a rough guide, the standard chest X-ray is 5–10 millirads (radiation absorbed dose). As a general rule of thumb, avoid X-rays unless essential and so minimise long term risks. Some parts of the body, such as the skin, absorb X-rays more easily than, for instance, the bones, which require a much higher dose and are therefore more questionable. If you want to know what is wrong, this is a risk that has to be accepted.

Sometimes dye is injected into a blood vessel to outline tissue. Any faintness or dizziness should be reported immediately to the doctor, who can reverse the process.

These are some of the more usual X-rays:

Barium meal In this examination the radiologist gives the patient a glass of thick, white and putty-like gruel, usually flavoured to help it go down more easily. It outlines the stomach (you may ask the radiologist to let you watch it passing through) and as it is not digested it leaves the body without trace. A barium enema is when the same substance is administered via the rectum. This is a lengthy and unpleasant procedure, though not painful.

Intravenous pyelogram (IVP) This is to discover if a tumour is interfering with the urinary system. An iodine compound is injected into a vein, to be studied as it passes the kidneys through the ureters and into the bladder. X-rays are taken to monitor the course of the dye. This is not a painful procedure and produces a rather warm sensation. It all takes about an hour and a patient should be able to get himself home afterwards.

Lymphangiogram This is a two part test as an in-patient —
lengthy and uncomfortable. It may help you to take an interest
in exactly what is going on, so ask for a step-by-step account if
you need entertaining. The purpose of the lymphangiogram is
to look at the lymph vessels and nodes of the legs and
abdomen. A small amount of blue dye is injected into the
upper part of each foot close to the toes and this is taken up by
the lymph vessels over the top of the feet. A local anaesthetic is
then given to freeze the skin and a small incision is made into
which the doctor injects a radio opaque dye that will show up
on X-ray. This is a slow process as the dye fills the lymph
vessels of the legs and abdomen.

You will need a friend or a good book to pass the time. It
takes about four hours, lying quite still. Afterwards, a few
people may turn a little green, while others feel as if they had
'flu. It's sensible to sit with feet up next day to prevent swelling.
The feet should be kept quite dry for at least 24 hours — contact
with dampness causes burning. Next day, be ready for more
X-rays and an IVP. Stitches in the feet are removed 7–10 days
later and there may be soreness and swelling for a time.

Arteriogram or venogram These are specialist tests to outline
an artery or vein and, again, involve the injection of dyes but
they vary according to the site of the blood vessel to be
outlined. They may be done under local or general anaesthetic.

Oral cholecystogram In this case, the dye is taken by mouth
(after the bowels have been cleaned out over two previous
days) and the X-ray is to look at the outline of the gall bladder.
There is no discomfort and no side effects, and the patient
should be able to drive home after an hour and a half.

Myelogram A myelogram is a lumbar puncture 'plus'. It is used
to X-ray the space around the spinal cord within the bony
spine. Under local anaesthetic, a thin needle is passed into the
fluid in the spinal canal and withdrawn. To turn this lumbar
puncture into a myelogram, dye is then injected and the patient
inclined, so that the dye runs down the canal; this enables the
radiographer to see if there is a blockage en route. The test only
takes an hour and is usually done when the patient is already in
hospital. It can leave a nasty headache but after a quiet period
lying flat, that passes.

Tomogram This is a specific way of homing in on a particular area and focusing on abnormalities too small to be picked up during a normal X-ray. It involves swinging the machine in an arc over the patient, taking a series of films – known as cuts – and changing the film automatically each time.

CAT scanning (Computer Assisted Tomography) This is a revolutionary method of taking X-rays. CAT scanners are still few and far between, and hospitals on tight budgets usually have to rely on local voluntary funding to maintain them, once installed.

The CAT scan differs from a ordinary X-ray in that there is an electronic X-ray detector instead of the usual film and the X-ray source rotates around the patient. The scanner produces a narrow beam of rays and as it rotates around the part of the body under examination the detector receives information on its density. All the information, seen from all angles, is processed immediately by computer. The result is a series of pictures like slices through a cake which can be constructed into a three dimensional picture. Apart from a nasty liquid which it is necessary to drink, the scan is painless, just boring.

Radioisotope scanning Certain parts of the body absorb different chemicals (such as iodine which is taken up by the thyroid gland). By administering these chemicals in radio-active form – called isotopes – they cause a radioactive emission from the area in question, which can affect photographic material and reveal abnormality. These painless tests generally last about an hour and can be used for most areas.

Ultrasound Many women who have been pregnant will be familiar with this simple, painless procedure. The patient is asked to drink plenty of fluid in order that the bladder is full and a clear picture obtained. During the test, a special conductor gel is smoothed over the abdomen and the small round 'probe'. A torch-like instrument is then passed over the body, beaming sound waves and picking up those from the body, building a picture of the internal organs and revealing any disturbance. This echo is reproduced on a photographic plate. Ultrasound is effective on the abdominal cavity and liver. There is no risk, and it all takes about half an hour.

Magnetic resonance scanning This painless, new, sophisticated technique measures the water content of tissue. Cancer growths have a different water content and give off different signals.

Scanners

Walk around the notice boards of almost any town in Britain today and you will find details of jumble sales, sponsored walks, charity fashion shows — all organised by energetic volunteers to raise money for a scanner for the local hospital. It is a strangely British phenomenon. Nowhere else in Europe could this happen. In America, of course, hospitals buy them off the shelf like packets of soap. Britain has fewer scanners than almost any other western country.

The CAT scanner was a British invention — the brainchild of EMI's senior research assistant, Mr Godfrey Hounsfield (now Sir) in the mid-sixties. It was launched in 1972.

The initiative for a local Scanner Fund Raising Group usually comes from the public rather than the hospital and there are now about 120 machines in the country — that is, one for every two health districts. The hospital indicates which kind of machine is needed. Costs vary; the price of a new, low-priced version is around £220,000, compared with £1m for a magnetic resonance scanner (there are only 20 of these) and £50–60,000 for an ultrasound machine. Maintenance costs — and this is the rub — are way beyond the pocket of most hospitals. So Scanner appeal groups usually attempt to raise enough to cover costs for five years after installation too.

Is it worth it? There are those in the medical world who believe Scanner appeals are dishonest because the public in general doesn't understand their purpose. You cannot have a scan as a routine health check. It is used in diagnosis after cancer is already suspected and a tumour is probably well-advanced. The number of lives saved compared with the expense is, they claim, out of proportion.

Other Hospital Procedures

Endoscopy This is the generic term for a series of internal examinations which the medical text books rate as 'uncomfortable' — in layman's terms 'horrible'. They are the kind of tests which don't hurt but may require all your powers of relaxation, meditation, visualisation, self-hypnosis – or perhaps a very strong sedative. If you are usually nervous, better to be doped to avoid a punch-up with the doctor!

● *Sigmoidoscopy* is for the examination of the rectum and part of the large bowel. This is the least difficult of the endoscopies, apart from the indignity; it is quick and patients may drive themselves home afterwards.

● *Colonoscopy* A colonoscope can be bent to examine the whole of the large bowel with a special light that makes it possible for the doctor to see round corners, rather like driving around Alpine bends in the dark. The test requires a sedative and though patients can leave immediately, better to have a chauffeur than drive yourself.

● *Gastroscopy* The principle is the same as for the colonoscope, but this time the doctor is navigating into the stomach. It is usually an out-patient test, but some hospitals suggest staying in to allow recovery time from the sedative. Many people find swallowing the tube extremely difficult and the throat is usually sprayed with anaesthetic, too, to prevent 'gagging'. If you are a tense, nervous type, ask the doctor to step up the anaesthetic dose so that you don't remember anything.

● *Thorascopy* is a new procedure, done under anaesthetic, for examining the lung lining and taking samples for laboratory examination.

● *Mediastinoscopy* This is minor surgery under anaesthetic to see if there is cancer spread to the lymph. The result may determine if further surgery is necessary, or whether radiotherapy would be better.

At the Natural Health Centre

Geopathic Stress and Radionics

Telephones, remote control TV, even electric light – all considered once as dangerous magic – we now accept (maybe unwisely) as miracles of science. But there are other miracles waiting only for greater research funding to take their place amongst the accepted medical techniques. Amongst these are geopathic stress control, radionics and BER (Bioenergetic Regulatory Medicine). They have been understood for centuries, intuitively, by primitive man. We are only now realising some of this magic may have been based on truth. They are complex, interrelated and each is a variation on the theme of natural earth energy and its effect on our health.

Geopathic stress In a thesis to the International College of Oriental Medicine, Richard Creightmore explains:

> The surface of the earth is woven with a pattern of etheric threads identical in energy and importance to the meridians of the human body. These are responsible for the health and growth of the natural kingdoms of the landscape and any interruption to their strength and harmonious flow has a subtle but profound effect upon the health of the local natural life.
>
> In the British landscape this network has suffered disruption and scarring from railways and motorway cuttings, quarries, tunnels, buried gas, water and electricity mains.
>
> The resulting disharmony manifests as a lowered quality of local natural life forces often through the medium of so-called Black Streams. These are meridians of energy associated with streams of underground water flow whose yin-yang balance has been distorted in favour of excessive yin. Ascendence of degenerative over generative influences occurs in places directly overlying such streams.

At the Southampton Centre for the Study of Alternative Therapies, where the work of Dr Julian Kenyon is stimulating serious interest over a broad spectrum of medical thinking, dowsing is used to find Black Streams. It has been found that a patient whose bed lies directly over this negative impulse may be showing a variety of stress symptoms from restlessness to cancer. Moving the bed may not be the complete answer. But it can help a cancer patient, they say. Better still is the neutralising of the Black Stream by a range of techniques practised by dowsers.

Disease, according to eminent acupuncturists Geoffrey Faulkes and Antony Scott-Morley 'is always preceded by an electro-magnetic disturbance which occurs before bio-chemical changes'. The understanding of Black Streams is moving medical understanding nearer the realms of science and many people believe that electro-magnetic medicine is the medicine of the twenty-first century.

The study of earth radiation above these Streams and their

relationship with cancer began in the 1930s. German scientist, Gustav Freiherr von Pohl, a respected dowser, discovered a relationship between earth radiation and disease in plants and animals alike.

Generally speaking, natural thermal radiation is harmless but when it is obstructed and becomes negative it is bad. Herr von Pohl devised a scale from 1–16 and began conducting experiments. In the village of Vilsbiburg, Southern Germany, he mapped all the subterranean water veins above strength 9. He then analysed cancer deaths in the locality. All 54 people who died had their beds above a strength 9 conduit. Doctors were sceptical so he repeated the experiment in Garfnau, where all 16 people who had died over the last 16 years had had their beds continuously over Black Streams. The findings were checked and verified by the Central Committee for Cancer Research.

Despite this, the findings of von Pohl were ignored and forgotten. Not till 1970 did these theories again gain ground. A number of research scientists then said that the influence of the electromagnetic 'energy net' combined with that of Black Streams was a causative factor in the release of cancer. There are now a growing number of medical dowsers in this country whose focus includes this type of geopathic environmental stress.

Radiesthesia Radiesthesia is the 'up market' name for the ancient art of medical divining as applied for the benefit of the individual patient. It, too, is a means of harnessing and interpreting unseen energies. Dowsers are quite respectably employed today by some local authorities to locate old sewer lines, underground streams on building sites and even lost graveyards. Some use the familiar hazel twig – the *virgula divina* or divining rod – but at the beginning of the twentieth century a French priest, Abbé Mermet, discovered that with the use of a pendulum, he could not only find subterranean rivers but detect blockages in a human's blood stream. It was he who called this technique Radiesthesia.

Today, many radiesthesists have adopted a pendulum for diagnosis – shapes varying according to their use. The pendulum held over the 'witness' – some object associated with the patient – responds to questioning by swinging or vibrating in a number of ways. There is so far no scientific explanation of how it works, though it is known to be part of the 'sixth sense' and related to the homing instinct of the animal kingdom. That something happens with a pendulum, there is no doubt. Interpreting that happening is the controversial skill.

The pendulum is used first to diagnose the root of the problem in the patient – which organ function is weakest, which food is causing an allergic reaction, which trace element or vitamin is deficient, for example. The practitioner uses the 'witness' – a photograph of the patient, his signature, a piece of his hair, blood or nail paring – in order to focus the pendulum onto the patient in question.

Following diagnosis, the pendulum is again used to determine the appropriate treatment, which may include, for example, herbal and homoeopathic remedies, Bach flower essences, gem therapy or more orthodox prescriptions.

Radionics – The Language of the Waves Radionics is banned in the USA, many say at the instigation of the CIA. It does not appear in the *Oxford English Dictionary* and *Pears' Cyclopedia* refers only to Radiesthesia and the 'pseudo science' of radionics. Despite this, since its discovery by an eminent orthodox physician, Dr Albert Abrams who died in 1924, it has flourished in Britain under the watchful eye of the Radionics Association (founded in 1943).

What is it? In simple terms, radionics is an extension of the art practised by dowsers or water diviners. It is diagnosis and healing by remote control. According to the RA, it is 'A method of healing at a distance with the aid of ESP and specially designed instruments.' Man and all life forms are submerged in the electro-magnetic energy field of the earth, they argue. Within that, each life form has its own electro-magnetic field, which, if distorted, results in the disease of the organism. So every organ, disease and remedy has its own frequency. These are known to the radionic practitioner as 'rates'.

Radionics instruments have calibrated dials on which such rates are set, both for diagnosis and treatment. The practitioner again uses a 'witness', which is placed on the instrument which measures its rate, and is able to detect distorted energy patterns and blockages.

Originally, Abrams had discovered that if he tapped the body of a healthy person holding a piece of diseased tissue the sound produced the characteristic note of the disease and not the healthy body. It was very similar to the use of clothing, hair or other personal effects by shamans or witch doctors for harm or healing. Being a scientist, he went on to discover that by connecting the diseased tissue to wire on which he'd placed the equivalent of electrical resistances, he could measure their rate and distinguish between diseases.

Albert Abrams had detected cancer in his wife 10 years before she eventually died of it. Over that period, her blood spot readings had gradually intensified, although orthodox medicine found no tumours and she seemed outwardly well.

As in most other holistic diagnosis, the practitioner is insistent that the patient must be responsible for his or her own situation. The practitioner is at pains to explain the real nature of the disease and probable need for a change in lifestyle and a respect for his or her body. He does not offer a miracle cure and admits that for some people the method does not work. But there are many documented cases of patients cured of serious illnesses who had been abandoned by orthodox practitioners. They believe that as many as 85–90 per cent of illnesses are psychosomatic in origin and that counselling therefore plays an important part.

In Russia, scientists also discovered that live tissue emits ultra violet radiation which can be measured (see pages 36–7). One of the team said: 'We are convinced that the radiation is capable of giving the first warning about the beginning of malignant degeneration and of revealing the presence of certain viruses. This could be called "the language of the waves".'

Radionics practitioners train through one of five approved schools offering part-time courses. Some qualified holistic therapists – osteopaths, herbalists, homoeopaths – also use radionics as an additional aid and take a short course supplementary to their own skill. Equally, radionics specialists often make use of Bach flower essences, gem and colour therapies when treating patients (see page 133).

Help from: Radionics Association; Colour Therapy (for both see Useful Addresses).

Needling

In 1986 the BMA claimed that the value of acupuncture rested in its ability to relieve pain but that its curative effect was unproven: a sweeping judgement of a system of medicine practised by one quarter of the world. It has taken some 6,000 years for the oriental concept that medical knowledge should be used to prevent, not treat, illness to be appreciated in the west.

In China, there are two types of doctor: the Superior, skilled in preventive medicine, and the Inferior, skilled in the curative art. A twice yearly check with the acupuncturist is much like our routine visit to the dentist. It is used as a means of detecting trouble before trouble flares up.

In his 'traditional' training, the oriental physician learns that the body energies – called *ch'i* – are carried through 12 meridians – or *mai* – each identified with a vital organ and each, in turn, representing an emotion: joy with the heart, anger with the liver, fear with the kidneys, anxiety with the lungs and nostalgia with the spleen.

The purpose of the regular check is that with very sensitive diagnosis the doctor knows, in the case of cancer, for instance, if the energy flow is clogged or blocked, and can realign the *ch'i* by means of extraordinarily fine needles. It is much like diverting a stream. This is a very delicate skill demanding an acute, sensitive understanding of the spider's web interlacing of human make-up.

Not until the sixties and seventies did acupuncture really register in British minds, and then only because of sensational stories that a group of doctors took back to America after a visit to China. They told of major operations – even caesarian births – performed, apparently painlessly, without anaesthetic. The voodoo label has been hard to shift but as public disillusion with orthodox methods grew so did an interest in acupuncture and, with it, a greater appreciation of its role, not simply as a stunt procedure but an increasingly recognised branch of medicine in Britain. A few NHS hospitals include it in their practice and will allow an outside acupuncturist to treat a patient who wishes to blend the two systems, perhaps to help with depression or pain. It is accepted that needling releases an endorphine-like pain killer.

Acupuncture really straddles diagnosis and treatment; most

acupuncturists grumble that patients tend to go to them only after they have been abandoned by orthodox doctors.

The only full-time College of Oriental Medicine in Europe is at East Grinstead, Sussex, where the founder, Dr Van Buren, teaches and practises traditional Chinese methods. A number of part-time courses are available now in London and elsewhere for orthodox practitioners. But the fully qualified acupuncturist studies for four years, full time, and there is concern in the profession that these short courses are dangerous. 'Would you allow an acupuncturist who has done a weekend course in surgery to operate?' is a fair question.

Dr Van Buren says surgery is quite unnecessary; it is removing the symptom without correcting the cause. We have been brought up to believe in the skill of the surgeon's knife. Faced with a malignant tumour and a specialist's wish to operate, how dare we say 'No thank you'? That would be a tremendous step. When nerves are already taut the decision to reject the familiar and face the unknown, maybe against the family wishes, must come from deep within. It must not be urged under pressure.

It helps to understand in essence what leads to such a controversial belief. Dr Van Buren explains that tumours occur as the result of an overloading of the system with toxins accumulated through the years and reaction to onslaughts of various kinds such as shock, diet, pollution.

The attack begins at birth when, as usually happens, black fluid from the baby's intestines is not always immediately expelled by the midwife. This forms a basis of toxic influence from the start. Then comes bottle feeding, wrong diet, tinned foods. The modern practice of immunisation further weakens the defences by suppression of childhood illnesses intended to toughen the system. Measles, chicken pox and mumps are a natural way of expelling bodily toxins through fever and toning the immune system ready to cope with problems of later life.

Anywhere along the life line, body energies can become tired and their related organs weaken. But it is after the mid-thirties, when basic kidney energy declines naturally, that accumulated stress can cause a problem. This is why cancers tend to occur more commonly in older people. The tumour usually arises in tissue controlled by its specific organ. An acupuncturist treating a person with bone cancer would look for trouble in the kidney, or, if consulted in time, would pick up the threat of bone cancer from kidney disorder. This is why it is useless to remove the tumour since that is not where the trouble originates.

A first visit to the acupuncturist is very satisfying because it entails an extremely thorough examination. Be prepared not only for questions about symptoms but about your lifestyle, emotional and sexual problems, and diet. The acupuncturist will look at the lines on your face and the direction they run, your skin tones and condition, he will note your tongue colour and moisture, your breath, the way you sit and move. Most important and interesting to watch is the taking of pulses. There are six to each wrist, one each to the twelve meridians and it is through these that the acupuncturist detects where the mind as well as the body needs nourishment.

All the meridians are reflected in the eye: the degree of sparkle, literally, represents the condition, and eye diagnosis is an important part of traditional Chinese medicine. A word of warning. Eye diagnosis must be carried out by a practitioner who either takes photographs or, better still, uses a slit lamp which magnifies the iris 40 times.

The needling process is not in itself painful – not at all like an injection. Effects vary according to the chosen needle site and sometimes there is nothing to be noticed. Sometimes there may be a leap in temperature or a light-headed sensation – sometimes a reaction in a different part of the body, but it is interesting rather than unpleasant.

There are over 500 registered non-medically qualified traditional acupuncturists in Britain – and 600 doctors using acupuncture. A list of each is available from The Council for Acupuncture and the British Medical Acupuncture Society (for both see Useful Addresses; the National Council and Register of Iridology may also be of help).

Reflexology

The reflexologist believes, like the acupuncturist, in the release of blocked or unbalanced energies. But he sees this energy flowing through the body in 10 channels. Each channel relates to a specific zone which has its terminal in the foot where any physical or emotional trauma is therefore mirrored. Having discovered the source of a patient's problem, the reflexologist applies gentle pressure at the appropriate points and so also frees clogged energies. This is foot massage – and very pleasurable too – most of the time. There can be sudden, short bursts of intense pain which are curiously exciting, like the discovery of clues on the way to a treasure.

The reflexologist will take a preliminary case history but may not ask your symptoms – it is his job to tell you what is wrong. The blocked energy for which he is seeking as he manipulates and massages the toes and the foot itself feels like tiny crystalline lumps beneath the skin. The aim is to locate them first – and then to treat.

Because tension is very often a direct cause of blockage, patient relaxation is vital to the reflexologist and correct breathing an important part of the session. This in itself makes a reflexology session enjoyable and beneficial.

5
The Waiting Game

The tests are over. The waiting game begins and daily life takes on an unreal, almost theatrical flavour.

If there is bad news to be broken, the task of telling falls sometimes to the family doctor, sometimes to the hospital specialists, a horrendous burden for which they may be woefully illequipped. In that painful moment you each have your back to the wall, locked in a situation from which there is now no escape.

The Doctor's dilemma is whether to tell the truth. The GP may know something of home background – the strengths and weaknesses of the patient, whether there will be support from a partner, parents or children – for not everyone has a family

Stephanie Simonton

Stephanie Simonton, an American specialist in family cancer counselling, has an inspiring vision of family life in sickness and health. In her book *The Healing Family*, she suggests developing a family game plan. 'The sheer length of time a family lives with cancer means that an open, well-thought-out strategy is very desirable. When cancer is diagnosed, patient and family members are thrown into shock and confusion. Sitting down together to decide how to handle the following days helps pull a family together and reassures each individual . . . a family's strategy must be flexible enough to change over time as the patient's situation changes and as other members' needs change too.' For, as she says, this kind of illness has a ripple effect – from the time it is diagnosed, every member of the patient's close family is also in need of support and understanding.

to share the load. The hospital specialist knows nothing and all too often that shows. He is a technician, and technology has little time for emotion.

Most cancer counsellors say it is usually best to tell the truth to patients and spread the load – in other words, to include the entire family in the verdict and help them to create a warm healing environment. Of course, care must be taken about how much to tell young or elderly relatives – a distraught granny whose own capacity to cope is fragile could unwittingly add to the strain on an overstressed family. For their sake, it could be better to shield her, at least, from the news. It is strange that close relatives of the very ill are often cushioned from what they do not want to know by a protective blanket of unquestioning, unseeing innocence.

The way in which this unique drama is played out can determine what happens next. For even the most articulate and together person can be numbed, pole-axed by being told that they have cancer. There are so many understandable responses: each has a negative and a positive side. It is suppressing them that is bad and may be what triggered the illness in the first place.

• A refusal to face facts. 'It can't be true.' This is especially likely if there has been a delay over test results.

• Tears. There is nothing wrong with a good cry – it is nature's way of releasing tension.

• Anger. This, too, is better out than in and is not always the chair-throwing variety. There is anger that it can happen at all, guilt that it might be your fault, and that you are no longer in control.

• Depression. Feeling depressed is part of the process of coming to terms with the fact that you have a life-threatening illness. Facing this can be the motivation for change.

• Fear. Usually not of dying but of pain and the horror stories surrounding the way cancer can behave.

• Loneliness. This comes about because subconsciously family and friends often withdraw . . . no one knows what to say to each other any more . . . they are afraid of hurting, so say nothing.

• Defiance. This takes many shapes; a spending spree for goods that aren't wanted, test driving cars there is no intention of buying – or the very positive decision to 'take hold of life'.

Penny Brohn

' "How do you feel when someone tells you you have cancer?" I've been asked this question so many times it must be an area of considerable interest to a lot of people. I have some difficulty in answering it because the first thought that overwhelmed me at the time was that, regardless of whatever emotional response was welling up inside me, I must not let my feelings show. In true British style, I braced myself.

'Eavesdropping later on a conversation between my informant and the ward sister, I heard that I "had taken it very well". I had not, in fact, taken it at all well. I hadn't raged or cried. His management of my crisis consisted of a pat on the head and an assurance that he was very sorry. I was glad he was very sorry. I was pretty sorry myself.

'It was all reminiscent of when my parents died. If you cried, someone told you to pull yourself together. If you kept calm someone told you to have a good cry. Nobody knew quite what to do. The person who told me I had cancer did so as if he had never done such a thing in his life before and would not expect to do so again . . . it was a depressingly inadequate encounter.'
(From *Gentle Giants* by Penny Brohn.)

What Now?

Once the initial shock has subsided comes the cold paralysis and confusion. Books on cancer are not daily bed-time reading and few people become cancer-wise until after the event. Then who knows what to do or where to turn?

If possible, keep calm. Be practical. It is your body, your life. Listen to advice but try to remember it is your right to take or reject it. Think positively and look ahead.

First, check your facts. You may ask for a second opinion. Ask to see an oncologist (a cancer specialist) and take a tape recorder with you. Medical jargon is not easy at the best of times, and under such strain you may forget what you are told. Two people within one family can make different deductions from such an interview.

Helpful information will flood in from friends. They will

give you details of miracle cures, clinics at all ends of the earth
... success stories. Much of it will be impractical and
confusing – best to file everything in a business-like manner.
Keep control.

Decisions will have to be taken sooner rather than later.

Most people follow the 'safe' familiar path to the nearest
NHS hospital because it is the only option presented to them.
Many family doctors are unaware of the tremendous advances
in complementary techniques that are available, even within
their own areas. All too often if these therapies are known of at
all they are presented as an alternative to orthodox medicine.
Sometimes this may be the case but there should, at this stage,
be no such confrontation. There is an increasing awareness
within NHS hospitals of a need to heed the words of the
holistic doctors, and a few are prepared to work in tandem.
Sadly, the block usually arises at the level of the consultant
oncologist whose training has led him to refute any method
that cannot be scientifically proven. The very spiritual nature
of many 'fringe' ideas means they cannot be measured in this
way.

For many families, the choice is dictated by purely practical
facts. Travelling is a problem for the patient and his family.
Cost, too, is a stumbling block. Holistic doctors are few and
far between in some parts of the UK but, by nature, they are
compassionate and a sliding scale of charges is usually
possible. But even a sliding charge is no good if you are on a
low wage and there is a hefty train fare to get to the centre.
Transport is normally available to a State hospital, if needed,
but not to a holistic health centre, although there are
sometimes charitable funds available to help extreme cases.

There is also a question of trust. The ancient skills of the
alternative therapist are new to most of us in the west. Very
often cancer is the trigger which awakens curiosity in this area.
Sadly, too often the decision to try acupuncture, or a specialist
diet, is taken too late – only when orthodox methods appear to
be failing do we clutch at the alternative straws.

This is not surprising because it is hard to trust a man whose
qualifications you can't judge and whose skills appear so
intangible. So put the same test to your family doctor. You
probably acquired him, rather than chose him, when you
moved to your present home. Do you know when *he* qualified

or how recently his knowledge has been updated? Do you understand the medical expertise of your hospital oncologist? Will *he* tell you how many patients he has 'cured'?

This applies equally to all methods. In most cases there is a professional body or organisation you can consult for re-assurance – and *provided your chosen complementary therapist keeps in touch with your own family doctor, you cannot go far wrong.*

Who to Turn to

There are now more than 300 registered Self-Help Groups throughout Britain. They vary in size and in aim. Some are run in private homes for intimate discussion and sharing of problems in a club-like atmosphere; there are larger centres practising some therapeutic techniques such as relaxation, meditation and nutrition. Very often they meet in village and church halls and are nerve centres of information about specialist methods worldwide, about new research and the work of individual cancer experts, as well as offering day-to-day support for patients and their families. These groups are often run by sufferers with the backing of as many local doctors as can be drawn in.

In addition, there are the natural health centres and the specialist practices. These are usually staffed by trained practitioners and are the equivalent of the NHS health centres or group practices. They are still few and far between. Some specialise in cancer, others are natural health clinics with a cancer section.

Far from being introspective and claustrophobic the atmosphere in most Self-Help Groups is cheerful, positive and unselfpitying. There is laughter and total honesty. Even so, many hospitals have shamefully ignored and even been hostile to their work; there is a patronising and occasionally aloof dismissal of their existence. But there are now a growing number of enlightened hospitals prepared to encourage and house a support group within their own walls. They acknowledge the patient's need for community-based help from the moment of diagnosis. Much depends on the attitude of the oncologist.

St Mary's Hospital in London has a team working within the system which aims to build bridges between the patients and the nursing staff to whom patients so often turn when they are bewildered and need guidance. It has close links with the British Holistic Medical Association too. The principle on which the team functions is 'If I do it for you, I help you today. If I teach you, I help you tomorrow.' They teach meditation to cancer patients because 'Anyone can relax when the going is good. To relax in the face of pain is tough.' Hypnosis and psychotherapy are also included in the help available. They preach enlightened awareness of both orthodox and holistic methods, believing that quality control and ethical restraint are equally important in each, that orthodox medical jargon is as confusing to the patient as the wilder claims of some fringe practitioners. The efforts to help 'clients', as patients are called, are continued after discharge – no question that a cancer patient will find himself being told to 'Go home and sit in the sun', as a chilling euphemisms for 'that's your lot'. St Mary's care continues for as long as the patient needs it.

Nurses who see patients on a more personal and consistent basis understand only too well the need for such support and much of the pressure for a change in attitude is coming from them. The Royal College of Nursing itself is increasingly enlightened in its sympathetic encouragement of close co-operation between all those involved in the care of patients, family and friends.

Coordinating all this information and feeding it on request to telephone callers are three main national centres of advice. These are New Approaches to Cancer, Bacup and Cancerlink. They differ in their approach but none of them will tell you what to do – their role is to act as an information centre, the next step is up to you.

Cancer can occur in any part of the body – except the spirit.

Although it is possible to explain in clinical terms the symptoms and characteristics of each type of cancer, no written words can reflect the feelings, the pain and day-to-day ups and downs, the fears and emotions surrounding each individual case. No amount of explanation by a doctor or even a nurse can match the reassurance of sharing the load with someone else who is fighting the same battle.

All these organisations will help you to simplify the choices

Ivan Ilych

Tolstoy described the isolation of this time with painful insight. This is the kind of response that families must understand can sometimes happen, and should be extra patient and aware of the possibility.

'The pain in his side oppressed him and seemed to grow worse and more incessant, while the taste in his mouth grew stranger and stranger. It seemed to him that his breath had a disgusting smell, and he was conscious of a loss of appetite and strength. There was no deceiving himself: something terrible, new, and more important than anything before in his life, was taking place within him of which he alone was aware. Those about him did not understand or would not understand it, but thought everything in the world was going on as usual. That tormented Ivan Ilych more than anything. He saw that his household, especially his wife and daughter who were in a perfect whirl of visiting, did not understand anything of it and were annoyed that he was so depressed and so exacting, as if he were to blame for it. Though they tried to disguise it he saw that he was an obstacle in their path, and that his wife had adopted a definite line in regard to his illness and kept to it regardless of anything he said or did. Her attitude was this: "You know", she would say to her friends, "Ivan Ilych can't do as other people do, and keep to the treatment prescribed for him. One day he'll take his drops and keep strictly to his diet and go to bed in good time, but the next day unless I watch him he'll suddenly forget his medicine, eat sturgeon – which is forbidden – and sit up playing cards till one o'clock in the morning." ' (From *The death of Ivan Ilych* by Leo Tolstoy.)

now ahead. They will guide you through the range of treatment on offer from private clinics offering the theories of one man, the religious centres and the specialist hospitals.

New Approaches to Cancer

New Approaches to Cancer was the first of the national advisory organisations and is the only one dedicated, so far, to a holistic 'gentle' approach. The goal is cooperation, not confrontation, with orthodox doctors.

Based in the peaceful Kentish countryside, its administration staff is much smaller than that of the other two groups but draws upon the internationally respected expertise of such specialists as Dr Lawrence Le Shan in America and Dr Hans Moolenburgh in Holland. Director Donald Stevens says: 'We encourage people to look more deeply and to participate in working on their illness. However powerful the weapons of surgery, radiation and drugs, to attack the tumour alone is not enough.'

New Approaches aims to work alongside existing medical facilities so that patients and their families have the best support possible. They help the establishment of Self-Help Groups, run lectures and maintain a constant phone advisory service linking patients with support groups in their own area and supplying them with information. They also have an extensive library of cassettes and a video for sale or hire, which describes the holistic approach to cancer in layman's terms.

Help from: New Approaches to Cancer (see Useful Addresses).

Cancerlink

Cancerlink was founded in 1981. Its four founder members and the advisory board are mostly rooted in orthodox medicine though it will provide information about complementary methods when requested: officially, their attitude to alternatives is guarded. Its aim is to catalyse the formation of cancer support groups and to provide support for them on a practical and emotional level. They will train volunteers wanting to establish local cancer support groups. They also have an extensive library.

Founder Amanda Kelsey says 'Three out of five calls are about pain – that is the greatest dread and the area in which patients are most badly let down. There is really no need for pain in cancer today.' Amanda says that letters are hard to handle:

> So often people do not make themselves clear. They come to us saying the doctor says there is no more he can do and they are desperate. We try to give them a feeling of control over their own destiny. We are very anxious that patients should not become obsessed with an idea that does not fit in their own particular framework. Very often they need, for instance, the comfort and security of familiar goods around. An extreme diet would not work.

Help from: Cancerlink (see Useful Addresses).

Bacup

Bacup was born in 1985 with a fanfare of publicity surrounding its founder — a young but greatly respected hormone specialist at St Bartholomew's Hospital in London. Dr Vickie Clement Jones was herself suffering from cancer, but her vibrant energy and medical contacts ensured that Bacup was extremely well-funded and organised from the start.

When Vickie was told, at the age of 32, she had ovarian cancer, she was angry, frightened and despairing. 'As a doctor and a patient I knew so little.' Her response to her illness was to plan an American-inspired, national information service which would feed anxious callers the kind of facts she had been unable to discover herself. She went to the United States, returned with several suitcases full of literature and began lobbying prospective funders.

Today, Bacup has a full-time staff of 14, a huge publications library, runs a glossy newspaper and answered some 15,000 calls over the last year. It has been supported by most of the main cancer charities. Vickie has lectured, travelled and made television appearances unstintingly despite long hospital stays and increasing health hurdles. Her sustained enthusiasm brought in £250,000 in six months.

The bias is strongly towards the orthodox approach. Though Bacup will give information, if asked, on complementary therapies there is a frank disenchantment, and often considerable concern, about methods which Vickie sees as giving false hopes and often dangerous advice. She is also concerned that the concept of controlling your cancer produces guilt if you don't. So Bacup is the source for all those committed to traditional methods, or needing to know about hospital treatments. A pilot patient-to-patient scheme has been started, and there are plans for a national counselling network and of crisis intervention centres.

Help from: Bacup (see Useful Addresses).

FOUR CENTRE PROFILES
Each of the following offers a different style of support; centres like these are opening every week and there are now over 200 in Britain.

Bristol

The Bristol Cancer Help Centre, opened by Prince Charles in

1983, was the flagship of the Self-Help movement. It is the best known, and has received the greatest exposure in the media. This is partly because, like all flagships, it was at the forefront. The ideas it pioneered appeared controversial and radical, but it was also because the Centre was inspired by the young, attractive co-founder, Penny Brohn, who was herself a cancer patient. She was articulate and phenomenally energetic and became a figurehead well able to put across a new message to cancer patients.

In 1979, Penny was told she had breast cancer and reacted by rebelling violently against the straightjacket of orthodox treatment. Her own personal response was to embark on a frenetic, globe-trotting quest for help from some of the great men in the world of cancer. She went to Dr Issels in Bavaria and to Dr Ernesto Contreras in Mexico, struggling with the spiritual and physical conquest of the cancer within herself.

In her book, *Gentle Giants*, she speaks of a process, not an event, a healing not a cure. She talks of 'growing up. Because this process didn't really start in me until I got cancer . . . it precipitated a dramatic reshuffling of my life and a rapid rate of change. You don't have to have cancer for this to happen to you. Any crisis will do.'

When she returned home some months later

> . . . our home was bristling with negative ionisers, orgone generators, water filters, bean sprouters, juicers, biofeedback machines and no smoking signs. I was longing to share all this with other people. It had been the most awful struggle to find out what I wanted to know about these things . . . nobody should have to grapple with all this, feeling as lost and lonely as I had.

Her way of sharing was to set up the Bristol Centre. With the financial and moral support of Canon Christopher Pilkington and his wife, Pat, it was a personal crusade. They secured a bank loan of £350,000 – the Centre is still funded entirely by private donations. 'We knew we'd been led to something marvellous and the angels were in charge,' says Pat.

Today, Bristol is still the only cancer centre with residential accommodation in Britain: there are nine rooms, four double. It has evolved into the kind of therapeutic healing centre that would be beneficial for anyone to experience, well or ill. The atmosphere in this very beautiful building, high on a hill above Bristol, is soothing and entirely non-confrontational. The aim is to guide each visitor along a path leading to other highways and byways, to help them find their own particular way of coping. Penny says:

> I don't understand how a doctor can go from bed to bed in a cancer ward treating each patient the same way.
>
> I do not want anyone to assume that because I did what I did this must be the way for them. It was right for me. There is no need now for anyone from Britain to panic into booking a flight to Bavaria or Mexico. The teachings of the wise men in these centres is available through many centres in Britain today for those who feel drawn to them. But enemas and fever days are not for everyone – and there are effective gentler approaches.

There is no confrontation intended between Bristol and orthodox medicine. 'If I felt a patient would find more comfort and security by following the orthodox approach I would advise them to go that way. I may disagree with what you say but I will defend to the death your right to say it.'

There is a feeling amongst the Bristol team that children require very special treatment and are best cared for separately: families are guided towards one of the specialist caring organisations. Even so, parents are welcome and given support to help them through their ordeal because, very often, they are suffering more than their children.

The visitor to Bristol today may either stay for a week or come for the day – preferably with a friend or member of the family. Families need to understand what is happening every bit as much as the patient. They arrive on a Sunday evening and, having first read the pack which is posted ahead, know exactly what to expect. They see a doctor and a counsellor for uninterrupted discussion – maybe the longest time they have had to pour out their feelings – and immediately the burden is lightened. They learn relaxation and meditative techniques: they learn nutrition and the value of vitamins. They can have spiritual healing and see a priest.

Food is home-cooked, pure and vegetarian, but the Bristol nutritional programme is not rigid and can be adapted. Patients are encouraged to learn how it is all done, on the spot, in the kitchen. 'Don't be too hard on yourself,' advises Penny, 'it's a bit of a struggle in the early days and it may be weeks before you get to grips with everything.'

Once in touch, the link need never be broken. There is a nurse available on the phone, day or night. Patients return time and time again. Some have been coming for five years, with hospital treatments in between. 'We'll help with that too.' They seem to develop their potency, to shift from assuming the role of the helpless victim to taking responsibility for themselves.

The Bristol staff are aware that there are many people who could never afford the cost of such a haven. They know there are residents on Bristol council estates who cannot afford the bus fare to the Centre. The weekly charge for accommodation, food and all treatments is £475, and relatives are charged £110. A bursary, for which funds are raised separately, can help to meet the expenses when there is real need. Even so, the Bristol philosophy and programme are available through many other centres around Britain: there are also tapes and a great deal of published literature, and staff lecture all over the country.

Help from: Bristol Cancer Help Centre (see Useful Addresses).

Morecambe Bay

The blazing sun, the waves lapping, the sound of seagulls and children on the beach – all pictures in the mind, soothing the stresses of cancer patients at the Morecambe Bay Centre. Once a month they come from as far away as Scotland – often 70 at a time – to share a day of meditation, relaxation, dance therapy and gourmet food cooked specially on the premises. Quality of life is the theme . . . the bee in the bonnet of Bea Vernon who started the group in 1983.

When Bea had a mastectomy ten years ago she took a leap in the dark – to holistic methods. She became involved in the launching of the Bristol Centre. There are no cure claims at Morecambe Bay, nor any attempt to replace chemotherapy or radiotherapy. Instead the aim is to strengthen inner resources in order to fight the disease with every possible weapon. Patients and their friends or relatives are divided into groups and take part in a series of half hour classes. They are encouraged to work on an individually planned programme of diet, counselling, breathing techniques, relaxation, meditation and other natural therapies. It is a direct, unemotional but immensely warm atmosphere which patients say leaves them with a sense of wonderful well-being.

Help from: Morecambe Bay Help Centre (see Useful Addresses).

Wessex Cancer Help Centre

The Wessex Cancer Help Centre was also modelled on Bristol and opened the same year – 1983. It now has a growing team of practitioners working with the volunteer centre staff. These include orthodox doctors, homoeopaths, psychotherapists and acupuncturists. There are also six chaplains. Emphasis is now strongly on diet and based on a blend of several approaches. There are some interesting and controversial theories, especially concerned with the toxic effects of plastic not only in food wrapping and containers but as a finish for paint and wallpapers. Could there be a link between the high brain tumour rate in children and plasticised mattresses in nurseries decorated with plasticised paint, they ask?

The Wessex Centre has a detailed and fairly formidable check list of what are believed to be cancer triggers – including washing up liquids (use soda), detergents (use soapflakes), parsley, celery, nuts, and much, much more. It is open to healthy people seeking preventive advice.

Help from: Wessex Cancer Help Centre (see Useful Addresses).

CYANA (Cancer – You are Not Alone)

The ladies of this group are practical and gutsy with their feet firmly rooted in the difficult soil of London's East End, and they have a determination to get a better deal for cancer patients.

They understand the problems of waiting for hours in the DHSS when you are sick, or struggling on the buses with a trolley in the rain when you've had a lumpectomy and you can't lift your arm. They know about diets and alternative therapies and invite lecturers to speak. The majority of members are using fringe therapies as a back-up to the national health routine. And they laugh a lot.

Five of the CYANA committee members must be cancer patients themselves – it is the only way to understand the true nitty gritty of what is needed, they say, and the reality of what you are facing. They run a 24 hour service on the phone and a drop-in day once a week. Men, they say, are not so good at self-help – they like to be directed.

Help from: CYANA (see Useful Addresses).

Vi Mitchell

Vi Mitchell finally discovered she had cancer by 'pinching' her medical notes from the doctor's desk and reading them in the loo. Up until that time, despite a colostomy operation, a hernia and then a painful lump in the groin which her consultant said he could not feel, no one had ever mentioned the word cancer. But there it was in black and white: 'metastatic carcinoma in the lymph gland of the groin' – and previously carcinoma in the rectum.

She had asked for the truth. 'But they lied to me all along the line. I was furious', she says. 'How could they underestimate me as a person like that? I might have died. I should have been given the chance to make arrangements.'

But Vi is not one to be defeated. This was eight years ago when she was 52. She had had a very active life as a single parent of one son, working in swimming pools, bars, farming, waitressing and globe trotting. 'I began to feel a gradual loss of strength – not even tiredness – everything was a burden. I had no pain and I might not have noticed anything if I had had a sitting down job.'

The first doctor said it was piles . . . the doctor in charge of her treatment disagreed and called for a biopsy, whereupon they said it was ulcers. A colostomy for ulcers seemed drastic, but she assumed they knew best. A year and a half later they removed the 'non-existent' groin lump and said it was to do with drainage from the previous operation.

When she discovered the truth, Vi's reaction was to become interested in her disease. She formed CYANA, one of the East End's very active support groups, and is now working 60 hours a week for them, fund raising, hospital and home visiting, attending conferences . . . doing all her own decorating, washing and boiling by hand with a cheerful disregard of her colostomy. 'I like to get out and about and see what life's all about,' she says.

She has switched to a specialist cancer hospital.

Ethnic Minorities
Many hospitals are sensitive to the problems of cancer victims in ethnic families, particularly women. There is, as yet, no centre where doctors are trained to understand the religious

and social beliefs that may, for instance, lead to a husband discussing his wife's illness with the consultant and making vital decisions without her knowledge. The demands of dietary regulations, too, can be a difficulty in hospital but there is a gradually increasing willingness to accept the special needs of these groups. The three main cancer care organisations — New Approaches, Cancerlink and Bacup — are all monitoring progress and will try to provide help and updated information for minority groups.

The Professional Bodies

The British Medical Association (Founded 1832)

The independent voice of organised, orthodox medicine in the UK representing some 75,000 doctors. Its aims are 'friendly and scientific'. A registered trade union, not affiliated to the TUC, it presents evidence on behalf of NHS doctors to the Annual Review Body on Remuneration, and helps with all legal aspects of medical practice. More recently, the BMA has assumed an outspoken pioneering role and has pressed for legislation on abortion, drinking and driving. For further information, contact BMA (see Useful Addresses).

The British Holistic Medical Association (Founded 1984)

Together with the British Association for Holistic Health and its associate members the BHMA is a tripartite organisation for all concerned in holistic health care. It has a membership of 1,500 doctors from all fields and specialities and associate membership is for the lay public. The BAHH is open to holistic health practitioners only. Work includes the organising of seminars and conferences, the education of doctors, medical students and allied professionals in the principles of holistic medicine and the encouragement of research. For further information, contact BHMA (see Useful Addresses).

6
The Major Forms of Cancer

The Central Nervous System

Brain

For relatives and friends, a brain tumour can be very hard to bear. Often, there is an even greater sense of isolation from the patient than with most types of cancer. It is fortunately fairly uncommon, and often not malignant.

Any tumour growing within the central nervous system — the brain or the spinal cord — is serious whether or not it is malignant. Because the brain, with its 10 billion nerve units (neurons), is 'mission control' any surgery can leave far-reaching and complex problems such as epilepsy. Any prognosis will depend on whether or not the tumour is 'encapsulated': that is, in a shell-like capsule, or whether it has roots invading the surrounding tissue which cannot be removed. Early diagnosis is essential, and it is not possible to determine if a tumour is malignant without surgery.

Symptoms are: headaches on waking, personality change, lack of coordination, vagueness, forgetfulness, that only the nearest and dearest may be aware of. Radiotherapy is possible for some tumours and supportive, understanding, post-operative care usually vital.

Both brain and spinal cancers are more often metastatic tumours with the primary site elsewhere in the body.

Spine

A tumour outside the spinal cavity is usually not malignant and can be removed. Any growth within the spine affects messages to the brain. It results in similar loss of coordination and communication, and can be very painful.

Gastro-intestinal Cancers

Pancreas

The pancreas is a gland lying below the stomach and alongside the bowel. It produces enzymes and insulin which are secreted into the blood. It lies deep in the abdomen and there are no early warning symptoms. Eventually pain in the upper abdomen, weight loss, loss of appetite and jaundice indicate all is not well. Because it is so difficult to diagnose pancreatic cancer, several of the usual tests may be necessary and the hospital may recommend an exploratory operation during which the pancreas itself may be removed.

Oesophagus

This is the tube connecting the mouth to the stomach. There does appear to be a direct link between this cancer and nutrition. Japan and Finland have a high incidence, whereas Japanese who live in America don't. Biggest offender is probably extreme diet or alcohol, especially if associated with smoking. The first signs are prolonged difficulty in swallowing.

Stomach

The incidence of stomach cancer is declining in the west. Its symptoms vary from a vague sense of feeling 'off' to acute indigestion, offensive and involuntary burping, and uncharacteristic irritability. Stomach cancer can be mistaken for ulcers and lie undetected, so those who want to know the truth should be sure to insist on expert judgement. The removal of part or even the whole of the large intestine does not, amazingly, affect activity or eating habits – beyond the need to eat more sensibly, little and often.

Liver

Primary liver cancer is rare in the west. It occurs rather more frequently amongst alcoholics and heavy drinkers and is believed to arise through exposure to certain chemicals such as vinyl chloride. Symptoms are difficult to pinpoint – maybe general weakness, loss of appetite and, possibly, abdominal discomfort. If the cancer is localised to one part of the liver, an operation may be possible. Radiation and chemotherapy may be given to control the disease but do not offer a cure.

Womb and Ovaries

Womb

Many women suffer agonies over symptoms that turn out to be fibroids. These are harmless, benign tumours that cause excessive bleeding and may require the removal of the uterus (hysterectomy). Any vaginal bleeding between periods or after menopause should be reported to the doctor. Usually this is harmless and dealt with by a D and C. Occasionally, though, a D and C reveals a cancer which can be treated by the removal of the uterus and is 90 per cent successful. A hysterectomy is a very drastic step for a younger woman if she is hoping to start a family. Uterine cancer occurs more commonly in late middle age.

Ovaries

The removal of the ovaries, uterus and Fallopian tubes can be 80 per cent successful when a tumour is found. Symptoms are undefined but include abdominal pain or discomfort, weight loss, nausea and possible shortness of breath. Treatment depends on the tumour spread and age of the patient. A young woman wishing to have babies may wish to retain one ovary and the possible risks should be thoroughly discussed.

Cervical Cancer

The prognosis for cervical cancer is good. It is easy to detect — although it does not always show up on screening until fairly well advanced. Latest findings suggest that it may be infective in origin and should be regarded as a sexually transmitted disease. Symptoms are an offensive vaginal discharge, bleeding between periods and after sex. Occasionally there is pain in the lower abdomen and bladder problems. Usually, a hysterectomy is the answer but in the case of a young woman, a cone biopsy only may be performed (the removal of a ring of the cervix) and the hysterectomy delayed until after childbearing. If this is done, regular check-ups are essential to monitor the state of the cancer. Radiation can also be effective for older women.

Breast Cancer

'Page 3' of the tabloids and the Venus de Milo represent the not-so-profound obsession both sexes have with breasts. That is, until there is a problem, when any woman will say she has become a neutered object of clinical curiosity. She is expected to forget her femininity and see herself as a car in which one of the components has worn out. Feminists may say 'So what'. But like it or not, history has conditioned us to be aware of, and sensitive about, the shape of our bodies. Breast cancer is not only a high risk disease: even if cured, it leaves psychological scars and unless treated sympathetically it threatens marriages, relationships and family life.

Even so, the attitude of too many doctors is still that of a pat on the head. A recent official study revealed, with masterly understatement, that 'as many as 25 per cent of women' need counselling after a radical mastectomy. One hundred per cent would be nearer the truth. Sad to say, many women grappling with the verdict of breast cancer have to contend with a curious lack of understanding and often cavalier treatment from male doctors. So don't be shy — be prepared.

There are 15 different kinds of breast cancer — you and your doctor should know what you are dealing with before planning action. Orthodox attitudes to treatment are changing. Do not allow anything to happen without full discussion, not only about surgery and its long term effects, but also alternative methods. What are they talking about?

The Radical Mastectomy

This is the total amputation of the breast, the fat under the skin, the chest muscles and the lymph nodes in the armpit. This inevitably inhibits the use of the arm afterwards and if the operation is only on one side can leave a patient with long-term balance and posture problems. There is very little proof that this drastic operation has better results than a simple mastectomy or even a lumpectomy. It is performed less and less.

The Simple Mastectomy

This is far from simple. It is a major operation still removing the breast but leaving the lymph nodes and muscles intact – and so greater mobility of the arm. This operation is usually followed by radiotherapy which is in itself debilitating, or chemotherapy.

Both leave your chest looking rather like that of a boy, without the nipple. The scar itself can be slight.

The Lumpectomy

This involves the removal of the tumour plus a wedge of surrounding breast. It is the least disfiguring operation of the three and statistically as successful. It, too, is accompanied by radiotherapy, or maybe chemotherapy.

Before any surgery be sure to list questions for the surgeon. Tell him if you would like to be considered for a breast-reconstruction operation which is now often performed during the mastectomy. Tell him whether you would prefer your scar to run vertically or horizontally. Ask him everything you need to know about the operation and your convalescence and after care. It will be extremely important to care for the arm on the mastectomy side; the hospital should help with exercises to get the arm moving (swimming is good unless you are having radiotherapy). Just keep your sights fixed on that day when you can again clap your hands above your head. There is quite a lot you will be able to do to help yourself. Simple things that are sometimes forgotten:

- Don't wear tight jewellery or sleeves
- Cover the arm in sunlight and avoid insect bites
- Wear a thimble when sewing to avoid open pricks
- Wear gloves when gardening, a mitt when taking food from the oven and rubber gloves when washing up
- Use an electric razor for safety – and be prepared not to be able to reach underarm fuzz for a while
- Treat any burns, cuts or scratches immediately

Apart from surgery, there is also a new and experimental technique.

Radium Implant

This is done under a full anaesthetic and involves the threading of a criss-cross of plastic-covered iridium wires around the tumour site, into which radioactive material is inserted and left for a few days. It is uncomfortable but not painful and leaves no scar. However, the implant can very occasionally be rejected.

Breast Reconstruction

Some hospitals are able to offer a second operation, usually two or three years after the original but increasingly at the same time, in which the breast is built up by plastic surgery. The techniques are improving but, even so, great care should be taken to think the process through before going ahead: some women would rather reconstruct their lives than their breasts.

It is possible to have the reconstruction whatever the size of the remaining breast, or if both have been removed. What happens? The surgeon implants a silicone rubber envelope under the skin and this forms a mound. The nipple, too, can be remade by skin grafts from other parts of the body. It is a most complicated skill. The total appearance will never be perfect but is, for many women, preferable to prosthesis.

The Story of Breast Prosthesis

Until the early forties, women who had had a breast removed were abandoned on leaving hospital to the hot sore agony of cotton wool or tissue stuffed into a bra. There was no alternative. Then came kapok-filled bags followed by inflatables which had a disconcerting knack of deflating noisily at embarrassing moments. After the war, Dunlop produced the first pear-shaped artificial breast. It cost a horrendous one guinea and was protected by patent for seven years. Everyone then jumped on the boob-waggon and experimental varieties in sorbo rubber and foam led on to the 'bean bags' of the late fifties. These were calico or linen bags filled with small plastic beads – they didn't burst, or leak, and they were much cheaper at about 2s 6d.

The first wobbly prosthesis that made any attempt to simulate the soft malleability of a woman's breast was the oil-filled, foam-back Trulife of the sixties . . . and it was a runaway success.

Meanwhile, back in his Bavarian laboratory, a scientist called Cornelius Rechenberg was not satisfied. He was sure a more lifelike and human breast replacement should be achievable. His first efforts were in fact plastic bags filled with wallpaper paste, but he persisted and, eventually, in the early seventies, the first silicone breast prosthesis was born. This was the immediate forerunner of today's styles. It was prone to bursting on aeroplanes but it led to a far more compassionate approach by manufacturers. Even so, ask any woman who has recently undergone a mastectomy what help or advice she was given by the hospital about choosing new boobs and very likely she'll say 'Not much'. Many hospitals have no prosthesis counsellor, are themselves ignorant of new designs and women do not discover there is a choice available on the NHS. Worse still, hospitals who will spend £100 on a surgical corset or £5,000 on a new leg, cut costs and will not spend £50 on a breast.

She is usually seen after her operation by a fitter – often this is a man – peering at her over a desk on which is laid a row of falsies. 'What size bra, dear?' he will say, handing over a padded prosthesis to put inside the bra she was wearing before. No concern for her individual needs, feelings or shape. She is left to face the world – and maybe the man in her life – with a sense of mutilation and shame. Nor is the despair felt only by the woman who fears her partner will not love her. For many single women the trauma is worse – doomed to a life alone, they fear.

This need not be.

The largest prosthesis manufacturer in Britain employs a product manager who travels the country lecturing, giving advice in hospitals, to women's organisations and Self-Help Groups. She carries with her a full range of all available styles from all the main designers, a job which, she admits with good humour, has its lighter side. Pity the security guard of an industrial company who insists on seeing the contents of her case! She encourages both men and women to forget their embarrassment, to feel and discuss the situation freely. She can help with the kind of questions that are so hard for a patient to phrase. Should I wear my prosthesis in bed? When should I let him see the scar?

Ideally, the facts about prostheses should be explored before the operation, preferably with a friend or husband. If a man is involved, so much depends on his attitude. If he can't cope, she won't. It is vital that he is involved in discussions, encouraged to talk with the prosthesis adviser, by himself if necessary, so that he can reassure his lady that she is still lovable and still herself: that there has been no change in her personality because she has lost an indispensable bit of her body. If he is worth anything, he will accept it.

After the operation much will depend on the extent of the surgery and the size of the lost breast. The weight of a prosthesis has to match the weight of the existing breast or there will be balance and back problems later.

On the ward she should be given a temporary prosthesis because the permanent form can't be fitted for eight weeks, or two to three weeks after the end of radium therapy. This is sheer humanity. A visitor's eye is drawn instinctively to the breast. Trying not to look is almost worse — better to make it comfortable for all concerned. No woman should be forced to look at her own scar until she's ready — it's best not to leave it too long, but the time must be right.

What is, then, on offer? The modern prosthesis is made to be worn in a bra of your choice (not wired). You do not need a mastectomy bra. It looks, feels and behaves like a natural breast so that your choice of underwear and clothes can remain unchanged. It is safe to swim in and must be washed and cared for just like skin. A woman is allowed a silicone prosthesis every two years on the National Health (they are guaranteed for one year).

Designs today are shaped to fit over the very varied hollows and bumps left by the different mastectomy operations. Very often when a lumpectomy, for instance, has been performed, hospital staff will assume that, since this is not an amputation, a prosthesis is not necessary. But a lumpectomy can sometimes leave a shrivelled, hard breast and there is a prosthesis designed to fit over it and match the shape of the remaining breast. There are also special designs for teenagers, and for ladies with naturally big boobs extra care is needed to counteract any one-sided weight loss. Many of those who attend private clinics can pay up to £200 for a breast that is actually available on the NHS.

The day of the first fitting is really day one of a new life. She is whole again and can start planning for a new dress, a date at the disco; she begins to feel more confident and can look forward.

Advice books and leaflets for mastectomy patients are necessarily clinically matter-of-fact; they fall far short of the sympathetic comfort any woman, married or single, heterosexual or lesbian, needs if she is to take a mastectomy in her stride. This is no time for modesty: do not be afraid to share your worries and experiences. There are a great many options open both in the treatment and after care of breast cancer patients today, and a great many sensitive groups to help both before and after surgery, but there is no substitute for a caring friend or the partner in a woman's life being involved in any counselling.

Help from: (for all female cancers) Women's National Cancer Control Campaign; The Mastectomy Association; The Royal Marsden Hospital Patient Education Group, (for all three, see Useful Addresses). Also: The Well Woman Clinics, part of the FPA, which is now a private organisation. Headquarters: Family Planning Association (see Useful Addresses). Your local Health Authority has its own family planning service on the National Health.

Lung Cancer

The story of lung cancer is, sadly, one of gloom and doom. Well over 40,000 people will die – mostly prematurely – next year from the effects of smoking. Some of these will be victims of referred cancer – caused by living or working amongst smokers. It is the most difficult cancer to contain and the easiest to prevent. Very often a tumour has already spread before any warning signs appear – when the cough, chest infections and swollen veins appear it may already be too late. The remedy: don't smoke, or be with those who do. Research shows that cigarette smoke produces free radicals – for up to five minutes after burning.

Lung cancer can take as long as 20 years to show. When you are 20 and enjoying a roll-up with your friends, 40 seems a long, long way away. Despite the fact that smoking is now a minority pastime, it is still on the increase amongst women and estimates from Action on Smoking and Health (ASH) state that by the year 2000 it will have overtaken breast cancer as the major killer of women.

There are two different types of lung cancer, each treated separately, but in all cases surgery is usually the first option. It is perfectly possible to live comfortably, if breathlessly, with only one or even part of a lung.

Small Cell Lung Cancer

This accounts for about one quarter of all cases. It is a rapidly spreading cancer which is usually discovered after metastases and so surgery is rarely performed; orthodox treatment is radiotherapy or chemotherapy or both. There is a high risk with lung cancer of a secondary spread to the brain and some doctors suggest radiotherapy to prevent this.

Non-small Cell Lung Cancer

This is a slower growing, slower spreading variety, and provided the tumour is localised in the lung, then surgery is more likely to be successful.

Help from: There is no specialist help group but The Chest, Heart and Stroke Association (see Useful Addresses) offers help to lung cancer sufferers. Advice on practical steps towards giving up or preventing smoking from ASH (see Useful Addresses).

Leukaemia

Leukaemia is cancer of the bone marrow or lymph nodes but appears as a blood disease in which white cells overwhelm red cells and platelets so that the body bleeds easily and is open to infection. Coping with its treatment demands fortitude and determination. There are major differences between leukaemia in children and that of adulthood.

In adults, there are two main types of leukaemia – acute and chronic.

Acute Non-lymphocytic Leukaemia

Most cases of acute leukaemia in adults are of this type. Early symptoms are general tiredness, skin bruising, gum or nose bleeding, or bleeding into the bowel or urine due to the absence of platelets needed for clotting. Ten years ago, there was no treatment and patients died very quickly. Today control is far more successful and patients do go 'into remission' for many years. But, because of the drastic nature of the chemotherapy involved, if the patient decides to go ahead, doctors should spell out quite clearly the effects it may have. In the initial stages, hospitalisation is usually advised. This phase is known as induction and involves high drug doses at a time when patients are already weak and ill. This takes several weeks after which the patient should feel much better and may well go into complete remission. This does not mean a cure but that doctors can see no further sign of the leukaemia.

Consolidation is the next phase – to knock out any remaining unseen leukaemia cells. Doses are still high but because the blood count is normal at outset, side effects are far less drastic. Maintenance is an experimental treatment with low dose drugs to delay any possible relapse.

Acute Lymphocytic Leukaemia

This occurs much less in adults than in children. It is treated in the same way as non-lymphocytic leukaemia, but the side effects are less horrendous.

Chronic leukaemia is, again, sub-divided into two types:

Chronic Myeloid Leukaemia

Although treatment is palliative, drugs do control this type of leukaemia and patients return to ordinary life. Chemotherapy is given orally with few side effects.

Chronic Lymphocytic Leukaemia

The elderly are the prime sufferers of this version of leukaemia and frequently the only symptoms are an abnormal blood count picked up during a routine test. Very often no treatment is given because it is dormant for long periods, and many patients continue living alongside it with little distress.

Hodgkin's Disease

This is cancer of the lymph glands. Unlike other cancers, it tends to occur in the young and in early middle age. In recent years, two major advances have revolutionised the prognosis for patients who would not so long ago have rapidly wasted away. Megavoltage radiotherapy and chemotherapy seem to have transformed this situation and, today, there is plenty of hope, especially if diagnosis is early.

Symptoms are drenching sweats known as rigors, tiredness, weight loss, itching all over, persistently swollen glands.

Bone Marrow Transplants

A bone marrow transplant is used when high drug doses of chemotherapy are harming normal cells or the leukaemic cells are no longer responding to treatment. Sadly, it is a carrot which is often snatched away. Quite apart from the problems of matching the donor and the recipient's tissues, the operation is delicate, sometimes dangerous, and extremely expensive. It requires specialist knowledge and should really only be performed in a centre with the appropriate back-up and laboratory team. Hospitals have become extremely worried about the amount of publicity given to bone marrow transplants since there are so few facilities available. Nevertheless, it does offer hope and is an option to discuss with the specialist.

Help from: Leukaemia Research Fund (see Useful Addresses). Founded in 1960, the Fund produces helpful literature and offers patients support as well as being the only national charity specifically concerned with leukaemia research. The Leukaemia Care Society (see Useful Addresses). The Society offers 'support in time of need, information, financial aid in cases of hardship and holidays in its own caravans.'

Head and neck

Tumours in the head and neck are rare but, since they can occur in a number of places each requiring specialist knowledge, their treatment is complex and unpredictable. Any tumour appearing in the ears, salivary glands, air and food

Christine Piff

The first thing you notice about Christine Piff is that she can smile like anyone else. In fact, her face lights up as she talks. This is remarkable because much of Christine's face was removed and the sight of an eye lost in an horrendous cancer operation seven years ago. Her effervescent good humour through the pain and dreadful disfigurement makes Christine a shining example of the uncrushable human spirit.

Christine Piff had been blissfully married for fourteen years and was completely happy with life as mother to three children and supervisor at their local playgroup when she first noticed a soreness in her face. The soreness became a pain, the pain proved to be cancer and her world was shattered.

The story of the next few months is one of tremendous courage and complete trust in the amazing technological skill of the hospital team. She lost her eye, half her palate, jaw and teeth too; was fitted with an obdurator and later a prosthesis to replace the missing cheekbones and eye; she lost her hair and had to re-learn to eat, drink and even to talk. 'Today I'd rather be seen with no clothes on than without my prosthesis', she laughs.

But Christine more than survived; she has achieved the almost unimaginable – being able to laugh with her family at the problems she grappled with. In the process she came to realise there were many other people like her with terrible facial disfigurements hiding, afraid and alone. So she started a network called 'Let's Face It' to help sufferers all over Britain and to provide a forum for sharing their heartaches and pain and to help them face the world. 'You can say things in such a group you would never say to an individual and you know they will understand. People tend to assume anyone with facial disfigurement is mentally retarded and even a district nurse finds it hard to accept.'

After all that, Christine can still say 'I have life, love and friendship. What else matters?'

Information from: Let's Face It (see Useful Addresses).

passages, nose, sinuses, nasopharynx, lips, oral cavity, tongue, tonsils, pharynx, larynx, neck, thyroid and parathyroid glands and gums come within this category. The brain and oesophagus are considered separately.

This is not a job for the local general hospital; team consultation and specialist care are essential. Symptoms depend on the tumour, but, in general, unhealing sores, difficulty in swallowing, sore throats and lumps should all be checked if persistent. Very often, they are spotted by the dentist during a routine visit.

Because surgery for head and neck cancers can lead to distressing disfigurement, they demand tremendous courage and the will to overcome. Fortunately, very few patients are confronted with this kind of challenge, but the story of Christine Piff is worth telling as an inspiration to all cancer sufferers.

Larynx

Laryngectomy means either the partial removal of the larynx, in which case the voice will be preserved, or, if radiation is not successful as it is in 90 per cent of cases, the removal of the voice box itself. It leaves a stoma – a hole – in the throat covered by a small plastic cap. Even then, with fighting spirit and plenty of support it is possible to recover the power of speech, if not like Richard Burton then maybe with a touch of the Mae West or Boris Karloff.

Joe Block, retired milliner and chairman of the National Association of Laryngectomee Clubs, had his operation 14 years ago and today he lives alone and travels the country lecturing on their behalf.

It is a hard task because the public know and understand so little and are embarrassed, but I urge every cancer patient to remember that we go into hospital as normal people and we come out as normal people. It is only the sound mechanism which has changed.

Recovering speech is easier for some than others but it can be done and whether you come from Yorkshire, Scotland or the East End of London, the new voice will retain much of the accent which made you 'you'. Sometimes, but not always, the sense of taste and smell is impaired.

Life for the laryngectomee is becoming increasingly better

supported. There are now special prostheses which make swimming safe and new developments are near completion which will speed up patients' progress towards a better quality of speech. Cancer of the larynx is more common in men than women. Symptoms are hoarseness, a lump in the throat and noisy breathing. Benign growths may re-occur but can be removed again with no ill effect.

The National Association of Laryngectomee Clubs has branches in many parts of the country whose aim is to help patients and their families grapple with the practical and emotional aspects of daily life. They work closely with speech therapists who are now always geared to the particular problems of the laryngectomee.

Help from: National Association of Laryngectomee Clubs (see Useful Addresses).

Prostate

Many men in later life have the routine operation to remove the prostate – the gland at the base of the bladder just in front of the rectum. This does not mean they have cancer. Because this is a very slow-growing tumour, many men who do not suffer from prostate trouble die of natural causes without ever knowing they had cancer at all. For this reason, prostate cancer in elderly men is sometimes left rather than performing a lengthy operation which could be even more dangerous than the growth itself. Symptoms are almost always a difficulty in passing urine – which becomes worse – difficulty in emptying the bladder, pain when going to the toilet, pain or blood when passing urine and the need to get up in the night. Removal of the prostate can cause loss of sexual potency; sometimes radiotherapy – which does not – may be as effective as an operation.

Testicle

This is one of the 'youthful' tumours, appearing rarely but more often in men between the ages of 15 and 40. It has two names: seminoma, the less malignant, and tetratoma, which spreads via the lymph or the bloodstream and is more difficult to handle and may affect fertility. If testicle cancer is suspected, a biopsy through the scrotum wall should *not* be done as this spreads the disease. Testicular tumours are removed through the groin or treated by chemotherapy and have a good prognosis, but the possibility of infertility arising from treatment should be thoroughly discussed.

Penis

Cancer of the penis is rare and occurs much more often in later life. Symptoms are erections not accompanied by sexual desire, pimples at the tip and bleeding. Orthodox treatment is usually removal of the tumour by surgery, if radiotherapy is not successful.

Skin (Basal Cell, Square Cell and Rodent Ulcers)

An unexpected spin-off from the package tour boom means skin cancer has become the most common – but the easiest to treat – of all cancers. It is the price we pay for the twentieth-century obsession with a golden tan.

Because it can be seen, it is simple to detect, appearing in the form of a bleeding or suddenly growing mole, a thickening of the skin or scaly patches. Fair skins are more at risk than those which are naturally dark. There are some pre-cancerous conditions that do not need immediate treatment but should be watched. Warts, ganglions, cysts and fibromas are not cancers, nor are tattoos in any way to blame for its development.

Malignant melanoma affects fair haired, freckled skins most and is more dangerous because, unlike other skin cancers, it spreads rapidly. Treatment of skin cancers varies but skin grafting techniques are now so good that disfigurement is not always a threat.

There are some simple precautions that can be taken against skin cancer. Limit sun bathing in direct light – especially if you are on the pill or taking medicine that is photosynthesising. These include diuretics for high blood pressure, anti-diabetic drugs, some tranquillisers, saccharine, deodorants, many aftershaves or perfumes. All these contain photosynthesising ingredients that intensify the effect of ultra violet light. Sun tan lotions do no harm, nor does touching or swimming with a person who has skin cancer.

Eye Cancer

Curiously, eye cancer may be generated by loss of ultra violet to the eye, and increases where sunglasses are habitually worn. It did not exist in Africa until tribes began replacing shady head-gear with trendy western sun-glasses.

Bladder and Bowel Cancer

Bowel Cancer

Cancer of the large colon is usually linked with the western diet which does not include enough roughage and so allows food to pass more slowly through the colon. If bowel transit time is prolonged there is a cancer-inducing bacteriological change.

Symptoms are constipation, blood in the stools, lower abdominal pain, unexplained anaemia or persistent change in bowel habits. If the tumour is confined to the bowel lining the chances are very good: if it has invaded the bowel wall, less good; less good still if it has reached the lymph nodes. The colostomy operation (when the entire colon is removed) is being performed less and less, and techniques of rejoining bowel sections are improving.

Bladder Cancer

The most common of the urinary tract cancers. It usually occurs in later life and is more common amongst smokers. Blood in the urine is a first warning, but constant trips to the loo should never be ignored either. It can be tackled with radiotherapy, but surgery is often recommended.

Orthodox treatment for these tumours sometimes, but not always, entails an ostomy operation. There are several varieties of ostomy but all mean the creation of a new passage for the discharge of body wastes through an opening in the abdomen. Sometimes the rectum is removed. The opening is known as a stoma – the Greek word for mouth. When the cut end of the colon is brought to the surface the operation is known as a colostomy; occasionally this can be a temporary arrangement. When the cut end is the ileum, the operation is known as an ileostomy. Urostomy is the name given to a urinary diversion. All three discharge faeces or urine.

It is hard to imagine laughter in the face of such a personal and potentially embarrassing form of cancer. Yet the ileostomy clubs abound with dignified humour. Our lifetime conditioning to the idea that there is something 'dirty' about natural bodily functions makes the prospect of discussing such private things with strangers, be they doctors, nurses or fellow sufferers, an agonising prospect for most men and women. Yet there are 100,000 people in Britain today who are ileostomists, colostomists or urostomists and no one but they would know. It's not fun. They would prefer to be as they were, but they do swim, play games, work, make love, have babies.

Having said that, there are many problems which face the ostomy patient and for which they are very often not prepared in hospital. Check that there is a stoma nurse, to help and comfort throughout.

First among worries is a loss of sex drive and a worsening of relationships. This applies more to men than to women, and especially to the gay community for whom there has been scant understanding. It is absolutely essential that these very sensitive questions be talked over because there are ways of learning to adjust, new ways to love, but without a compassionate and wise guide they are hard to find.

The practical aspects of ostomies, such as infection, soreness and odour, are also very hard to cope with. There are often complications with the stoma care itself as well as in the day-to-day management of the bag. All too often there is not enough advice on diet – simple warnings about asparagus, which produces a pungent odour, and the need to drink fruit juice, which has the reverse effect – would make so much difference to the early experimental days.

None of these distressing worries needs to be tackled alone. Anyone facing an ostomy operation would be well advised to go to one of the specialist advice groups *before* it is done.

Abbott Laboratories in Kent, where many of the wide variey of appliances are designed and manufactured, run a Stoma

Advisory service which provides counsel, puts patients in touch with experts in their own area and books which explain exactly what to expect. Before contacting them, you should try to face exactly how much you *want* to know. Their literature varies from the gentle 'soft' approach to the truthful, factual and explicitly illustrated variety, which is not always easy viewing.

Help from: The following organisations offer help of various kinds; all are listed in Useful Addresses. The Colostomy Welfare Group; The Ileostomy Association of Great Britain and Ireland; The Stoma Advisory Service; The Urostomy Association; Wallace Kingston Trust for Abdominal Diseases.

7
Action Stations

Anyone with severe illness who doesn't have a physician is a damned fool. He is trained to evaluate symptoms appearing or disappearing.

  You don't have to do what he tells you but you must have that advice or you are blind.

Lawrence Le Shan

Choosing Your Hospital

In theory you have a right to be treated in a hospital of your choice. In practice, that could land you far from home, bereft of visitors and isolated from your GP. There are, however, points to consider that may help you decide.

● A general hospital may be well endowed with specialists but not necessarily a cancer specialist – an oncologist – they are still a fairly rare breed.

● Specialists move around – you may have been given the name of a 'top man' in your area and it's worth finding out if any of the hospitals he works in is near to your home.

● How long are the waiting lists?

● Find out what specialist after care is offered.

● Is there a cancer care group within the hospital?

● What is the doctor's attitude to Self Help Groups?

Help from: National Consumer Council (see Useful Addresses).

Going to Hospital

For many patients, that moment when a tag is fixed on the arm means a loss of identity – de-personalisation. Their only defence is to hang on to individuality in any way they can.

Hospital is a world apart. Those who work there can become as institutionalised as their patients. Insular, competitive and rigidly secretive, there has in the past been very little internal communication between consultant and doctor, doctor and nurse. But as patients have become more self-assured and more knowledgeable about cancer, and nurses have found themselves at the blunt end of the questions, the need for change has become acute.

Doctors and nurses are seldom trained together. Communication is a soft option on the medical school syllabus — perhaps because so many doctors believe they are naturally good communicators. For any seminar or lecture on communication you will find one in ten doctors attending whilst there is a queue of nurses willing to learn. This breeds resentment, and doctor bashing is a currently sad reflection of the unease between them. The nurse all too often feels she is

---

Ted Jones

As a public relations man, Ted Jones says his work 'attracts worry like an Exocet to its target.' So when, three years ago, he was told he had cancer of the bowel he was too busy to think much about it. He carried on planning major campaigns and forgot about his illness.

But hospital, he found, was a 'cosy sanctuary from all the frenetic worries with which I'd erased my fear of cancer. I had nothing left to worry about so I turned to the alternative — curiosity.'

Taking a journalist's interest in daily life in the ward, he became engrossed in the soap opera events that followed instalment upon instalment, which also helped him keep cancer in its place. It was fascinating stuff and he even managed to write a light-hearted script for *Woman's Own* to pass the time.

The operation was a success. He's been frantically busy ever since and there has been no more trouble. 'Worries are native to living,' he says, 'so I made cancer the least of mine. The best way to survive is simply not to give up the ghost. That's the way to become one.'

the pig in the middle. She is with the patient most of the time, she understands the needs; she knows what the doctor knows but must not act independently.

Cancer patients vary enormously in their responses. Some need to know what to expect. Many want to be involved in their treatment and this should be regarded with respect. A few ask nothing and most doctors will take this as a sign not to tell. Needs change and doctors should listen to the nurses' sensitive monitoring of these shifts of mood. Communication in itself is neither good nor bad, but it must be individual and appropriate and two-way.

Hospital can make any adult childlike, totally taken over by doctors who 'know best', stupid and powerless, and this leads to depression. Serious discussion is not encouraged — everyone is conditioned to talk about the weather, local gossip, sport, to trivialise, to fade away from the importance of the patient's own life and so help everyone to keep the rules.

The consultant and his team sweeps in. 'And how are we today?' You don't know who he is. He doesn't use your name. He talks as if you don't exist and sweeps out for a huddled conference outside your drawn curtains. He may be a master of phrases you'd rather not hear. You are right to resent the pat on the head technique. He talks of 'your sort of illness', 'abnormal cells'. Doctors know the patient is scared and are afraid he may freak out. 'It won't mean anything to you.' 'Your liver's beautiful.'

Remember:

- The best doctors in the world can't make a person better unless the patient is in there, helping.
- Many doctors are themselves afraid of death and have not come to terms with their own mortality.
- Don't be intimidated. Make a list of questions, keep them brief and, if necessary, hand them to him for reply. Take nothing for granted.
- You do not have to make instant decisions. No surgeon should be given carte blanche to continue removing organs just in case the cancer spreads. It is possible to know beforehand exactly what is needed and discuss it.
- To the cancer patient helpless in bed, the nurse is a guardian angel; she is the messenger of life and death. But, with courage and her help, it is possible to bridge the communication gaps

and not to allow the powers-that-be to upset you. Understanding their situation helps a bit and good humour can do the rest.
● Ask for a time table of events in your day – injections, tablets, visits – it helps you to share the organisation of your life and understand the system.
● Ask the consultant what can *we* do to tackle this illness. Get in on the act.
● Invite him to sit on your bed. Find out his name and use it. Make sure he knows yours.
● An argumentative patient is labelled as a bad and difficult patient. Don't let that put you off. We pay £18 per family per week for the National Health – we do have some right of courteous reply.

There are ways, too, to keep links with the outside world. Ask your own hairdresser to come; if you feel capable, keep up some local club work. If you don't, then let the hospital staff know you feel rotten, and need to be cosseted. Says Stephanie Simonton, 'A patient who asks for the vulnerable part of himself to be recognised in this way is still assuming responsibility for his need by the fact of making the request. This is quite different from being infantilised by institutional settings because he has *asked* to be nurtured and taken care of.' The more politely assertive the patient, the better he tends to do.
   Once cancer has been diagnosed it is important to determine how far it has spread. This process is called staging. The course of treatment to be followed depends on the 'stage' reached. The main aims of staging are to estimate:

● How large is the original tumour
● Whether the tumour has spread to nearby lymph nodes
● Whether the tumour has metastasised.

Sometimes staging is carried out simultaneously with the initial tests, sometimes it involves more extensive procedures.

Surgery

> The most advanced surgeon cannot heal a surgical wound. He brings the edges together and nature heals.
>
> *Lawrence Le Shan*

Patients were not the only people to be knocked out by the discovery of anaesthetics in 1846. This, combined with the contribution of Joseph Lister of antiseptics, revolutionised the surgery scene. Doctors, too, became mesmerised by their new skills and the knowledge that now they could go where no man had been before. Surgery was by no means new. The Roman doctor, Celsus, had performed radical mastectomies but the suffering was horrible and many patients died. In 1718, Lorenz Heister produced his intricately illustrated *Chirugie* — a treatise on surgery in which mastectomy procedures had hardly changed in 1,000 years. It was not surprising that with the technical boundaries so greatly increased, medical men became more and more interested in the mechanics of the body as a machine. This is when they lost touch with the truth that the tumour was *not* the disease. Its removal could never ensure the end of cancer unless the underlying causes were removed too. With the pain of surgery and the danger of infection minimised, the death rate dropped.

Surgery today is probably the most widespread and successful of the orthodox techniques for tumours that have not metastasised. It is a finely balanced procedure; the removal of too much healthy tissue can lead to complications, the removal of too little will lead to spread. In all surgery there is inevitably an element of trust for even the surgeon can never be sure of its outcome.

There is no reason why you should not apply the 'Would you buy a used car from this man?' test. After all, this is a matter of your life and death.

Lasers

Laser surgery for invasive cancers is still at a very experimental stage. It is used as a temporary, palliative measure for bronchial tumours but comes into its own for the treatment of pre-cancerous conditions of the cervix. Unfortunately, the equipment needed is expensive and not generally available within the NHS. The laser is particularly effective because there is no cut and, therefore, no rush of blood to the site which can, it is feared, cause the disease to spread.

'A funny thing happened on the way to my stoma' Music hall jokes about 'my operation' may wear a bit thin but there is tonic and comfort in such exchange of experience: the confidence that comes with knowing you are not alone and can

enjoy the freedom of total honesty. Especially in general hospitals, cancer patients can still feel utterly desolate. Gall bladder and prostates are OK subjects – mention cancer and it can freeze a ward.

It's probably only in the gossip-swapping Cancer Support Group that you will hear colostomy patients talk, for instance, about alternatives to the dreaded colostomy bag. 'Use a pad – it works if you are passing stools.' They may air the problems of disposal from a tower block, if a patient uses 60 pads a month (at £1 a time cost to the NHS). They may grumble about the commercial bandwaggon surrounding cancer: is there a need for the plastic bags (such as those developed on the space shuttle) *and* the pad to attach to the stoma to prevent soreness, *and* the bag to go over the bag so that there's no plastic next to the skin, *and* charcoal deodorising bags, all of which 'make work for the working man to do'?

Such talk may seem strange when you are fit and well but ask any cancer patient and you'll find this team spirit is uplifting. It's practical too. The radiotherapy nurse may warn a patient that the area of treatment should be kept dry, but it's among friends you discover that damp air and bath steam can burn too; that African hair doesn't always grow the same colour after chemotherapy, that after a lumpectomy you can't easily brush your hair and that strap hanging on the tube is out. . . . On the positive side you learn of all the extraordinary feats of courage and achievement by both men and women that can be accomplished on the road to survival.

Radiotherapy

An invisible mist of radiation wafts in from Chernobyl and we are afraid of cancer. Men in white coats suggest radiotherapy to blitz a tumour and we clutch gratefully at straws. What is the difference? How can the same source kill and cure?

Natural sources account for 87 per cent of man's exposure to radiation. Flying in an aeroplane or playing the remote control of the TV set increases this exposure, as does living in a granite house in a place such as Aberdeen which is built on granite rock. Our bodies learn to adapt.

To Australian aborigines and North American Indians, land

overlying uranium deposits was an especially sacred power centre. These were the places to which the shaman or witch doctor went to become spiritually aware. Uncontrolled, as in nuclear disaster, radiation can be destructive and initiate the process that leads to cancer – or it can be directed consciously and harnessed for benefit by a priest or by a doctor in a homoeopathic way to attack the cancer itself. Very few radiotherapists or radiologists in hospitals appreciate the power of the tool in their hands. Theirs is a modern application of ancient wisdom.

Only a few fanatically fringe practitioners reject radio-therapy out of hand. Most believe that it should, like, to a lesser extent, chemotherapy, be used in tandem with com-plementary therapies, and that any success with cancer, whether it be through the miracles of modern science or the lost arts of old, must depend greatly on the mental approach of the patient.

In the Simonton book *Getting Well Again*, they say:

It is important to visualise your treatment as a friend and an ally. Our patients frequently report reduced side effects as a result of changing their attitude in positive supporting directions. For instance, one patient who feared his treatment began calling the machine giving him radiation 'George'. He held mental conver-sations about all the things the treatment was going to do for him. In addition, the patient made efforts to engage the doctors and nurses in friendly conversation, which included thanking them for their efforts. Shortly after this change in attitude, he began to experience fewer and fewer side effects. Personalise your treat-ment. Make it a helpful friend who is working with you to overcome the disease.

That's all very well. Radiotherapy can, in practice, be a lonely and awesome experience: one small human being, alone in a roomful of science fiction. There's machinery that is unseen, penetrating the most secret parts of the body and altering its basic structure. Why does everyone else withdraw? Why does it make the patient feel so rotten?

The story of the medical X-ray is relatively brief. Soon after its discovery by Wilhelm Roentgen in 1895, doctors realised it could cause or cure cancer. Precision X-rays – that is, those used to pin point and isolate the area of the tumour – is an even newer skill and until recently was more widely used in Europe than in America.

Beams of energy, known as X-rays or gamma rays, are given off by radioactive substances such as cobalt, caesium, iridium or radium, which are either kept in the machine which delivers these rays to the patient or in a small container which may be inserted in a body cavity (such as the uterus) or directly put into the tumour by needle implant.

This can be effective in two ways: for early tumours which can be shrunk or destroyed, or for secondary spreads as an addition to surgery in order to slow down their symptoms rather than effect a cure. In some late cancer it is also used to relieve pain. Its purpose overall is to destroy cancerous cells and damage the blood cells that nourish the tumour.

Radiation works well on precisely defined tumours such as those on the lymph nodes and especially on organs that are best not removed – cervix, vocal chords and tongue. But it does, at least temporarily, damage surrounding tissue and can have a variety of disagreeable side effects.

You are within your rights to ask (if you wish to know) what level of radiation dose is to be given (see page 64). The doctor may be surprised but should respect your interest. The higher the dose the shorter the period of time it should be given. Radiotherapy can sometimes involve daily visits for treatment for as long as a month, and if a patient has no transport or accompanying friend this should be discussed at the outset.

The most frequent way in which radiotherapy is given is as an out-patient, by a technician directing the X-ray onto an area previously marked by a blue cross. Jokes about that cross being in the wrong place are not always misplaced – if you think it is wrong, *say so*. Mistakes can happen.

In high doses radiation strips electrons from the body cells, altering their chemical make up. Lower exposures may have no immediate effect but may cause cancers in years ahead.

The unit of safety, in human terms, is the micro sievert, and the universally recognised danger level is 100,000 micro sieverts. One micro sievert means

- One tenth of the dose incurred by flying to Spain in a jet.
- The difference in annual dose from cosmic rays received by moving from a first floor to a seventh floor flat.
- One tenth of the average dose from a single chest X-ray.

- One tenth of the annual dose from radioactive fallout in the UK in the 1980s.
- Two-thirds of the average dose to the UK population due to discharge from nuclear installations.
  (Figures from the National Radiological Protection Board.)

It is possible to off-set some of the side effects of radiation by mental exercises and meditation which can also improve the beneficial aspects of treatment.

Chemotherapy

The sinking of an American ship off the coast of Italy during the Second World War was, ironically, to prove a life-prolonging event for thousands of people in the years to follow. The cargo on board was deadly mustard gas and the sailors who died were found to have undergone a radical change to their blood. The gas had destroyed the lymph cells. This event led eventually to the development of a drug, a derivative of mustard gas, that is used today to treat cancer of the lymph nodes. The effect of mustard gas on the blood was first described by the Krumbhaar brothers after the horrors of the First World War, but their discovery was not followed through until 1946.

Only 30 years ago there were still no anti-cancer drugs. Today, there are many and new additions are being developed all the time, some as a result of cancer research, others as by-products of unrelated experiments and they are used to treat a wide variety of cancers.

They are designed to treat the whole body. The drugs poison the cells' ability to reproduce. One prevents cells from forming the proteins and enzymes that keep them alive. Another kills by disrupting one part of the cell division process. A third upsets the hormone balance in the patient and creates conditions in which cancer cannot thrive. But the problem is that drugs are not selective enough – they also attack normal cells – and success depends on getting the right drug balance to demolish more bad cells than good. It's a complex system which may well mean making a chemical cocktail.

In practice this means that if a patient is recommended for chemotherapy there are many ways in which it may be given and reactions are unpredictable. For some people the treatment is a torture, at times worse than cancer itself, but there are others who go through the experience comparatively unscathed and for whom life is prolonged and even saved. Only you – with all the facts in your possession – can decide if you are prepared to try. Chemotherapy is administered in three ways:

- By mouth in tablet or capsule form
- Intramuscularly – by injection into the muscle or beneath the skin
- Intravenously – into the forearm.

This can be undergone as an out-patient, but if the drugs must be given by slow drip or carefully timed, then it may be necessary to stay in overnight. Because of the large numbers of chemicals involved, the treatment is usually spaced out and given either weekly or monthly. It is a comparatively painless procedure in itself, although prolonged chemotherapy may make the finding of suitable veins difficult. There is no reason not to work if the patient feels up to it between sessions.

If there is a price to be paid, it comes with the side effects caused by the way in which the chemicals interfere indiscriminately with the cells and, in particular, tissue composed of frequently dividing cells – stomach, hair follicles, mucous membranes. Sometimes, too, if there is damage to the bone marrow, the body cannot properly control infection. Hair loss, nausea and extreme tiredness are the most widely known side effects of chemotherapy. But there are many others, depending on the drugs being used and the site of the cancer, and there are some reactions that vary also according to skin colouring. Western hair, for instance usually grows again once the treatment ceases and regains its former character, whereas African hair tends to become straight.

The possible side effects on children should be talked over in detail.

Chemotherapy usually lasts as long as is necessary, though it takes several weeks before doctors can tell if the response is good enough to recommend continuing treatment. Sometimes, the drugs are used over a long period of time to slow down the cancer spread, especially in cases where the disease is widespread – this can produce a remission, especially in leukaemia cases. Sometimes they are used as a preventive measure (adjuvant therapy) to prevent the spread of a primary cancer and may be given for life.

The hospital should – but often doesn't – forewarn a patient with any information they need to cope with the effects of their own particular treatment. If there is a problem, badger the local support group for the kind of facts you need. Best to get it all clear before you begin.

Hair Loss

This can be partial but may mean total loss of body hair for the period of treatment. Wigs may be provided by the NHS. It is sensible to choose a wig, hairpiece or toupée in advance and get used to wearing it so that the change is less of a shock. (If you have long hair cut it before the thinning starts.) Now is not the time to change colour! Go with a friend and if you choose to go privately to a wigmaker try not to count the pennies – cheap wigs look tatty. Go for synthetic hair: it's easier to wash, not so hot and it's cheaper.

Hormone Changes and Hair Growth

Women taking androgens may find their voices deepen and hair growth increases temporarily, with a corresponding increase in sex drive. Men on oestrogen sometimes develop breasts and lose interest in sex. Menopausal women may bleed, but all these symptoms should be talked through with the doctor involved before any treatment.

Sterility

Sperm count is sometimes reduced by chemotherapy, and so there is temporary infertility, but erections and intercourse are unaffected. It is wise to ask the doctor if sperm can be frozen for future artificial insemination if there is any question of wanting a family later on. A close and loving partnership can be an incomparable help to a cancer patient but, much as it is needed, it is often hard to sustain. Be understanding and don't let it become an additional pressure. Sterility can become a problem for both men and women, and there are often attendant psychological difficulties.

Infection
Because chemotherapy affects the ability of bone marrow to produce platelets which affect the clotting of blood, you should take care not to cut or injure yourself. It is probably wise not to plan sports or manual work. Avoid forceful nose blowing and use an electric razor rather than a cut-throat. If possible, try to live normally, allowing a little extra time for rest as you may well feel tired.

Chemotherapy can also lead to a low white cell count, which makes it hard to fight infection. Avoid crowds, colds and keep scrupulously clean. Sweating, chills, sore throats, frequent persistent sores, vaginal itching, oozing gums, bruising, long heavy periods – all should be reported to the doctor.

The Complementary Therapies

These are the complement to 'orthodox' medicine. They include therapies that present a total way of life, and remedies that are a part of that philosophy. First consultations start at around £15, depending on the specialist, but can be considerably more. It is always worth enquiring, if you are financially stretched, since the principle of 'Robin Hood' is often applied.

Anthroposophy – the Mistletoe People
Anthroposophy is a way of living rather than an antidote to dying: a gentle nurturing of the mind and spirit. Its disciples sometimes appear to float in a world apart from the nuts and bolts of everyday reality and yet have a practical belief in taking responsibility for life – and that includes paying what you can afford for what you receive.

Anthroposophy was founded by the Austrian scientist and philosopher, Rudolf Steiner, at the beginning of the century. He developed a passionate interest in the prevention and broadly based treatment of illness and promoted a belief in the healing power of mistletoe as an adjunct to the treatment of cancer. He believed in the perception of soul and spirituality as directly as we perceive material things.

Anthroposophical doctors are all medically qualified first, with an additional training from the School of Spiritual

Science in Switzerland. This has become very difficult, for orthodox training is now so far removed from the gentler, anthroposophical approach. In Britain, anthroposophical doctors are hard to find. The parameters of anthroposophy are fluid and use is made of homoeopathic, herbal and anthroposophical medicines, as well as conventional drugs, plus a strong emphasis on therapeutic baths, massage, nutrition, movement therapy (eurythmy) and a wide range of artistic activities.

Iscador Mistletoe is a mystical plant whose unique character has been honoured for thousands of years. It stands apart in the plant world, having its own independent identity and life cycle, its fruit ripening in midwinter and the shape and the direction in which it grows seemingly unaffected, unlike other plants, by gravity and light. All over Europe, and especially in France, mistletoe is harvested with tender loving care. Its preparation as a medicine is a complex, radical affair designed to strengthen the body's immune system. The male and female plants are mixed in a gravity-free centrifuge so that it remains biologically stable with its properties preserved. The uses to which it is afterwards put depend on the host tree – mistletoe from the apple is helpful to reproductive organs and the breast while from the oak, it is for the prostate.

According to anthroposophists, too, cancer is a 'cold' disease. It is a degenerative, hardening illness which could, they believe, like acupuncturists, be on the increase partly because we have upset natural human development by stamping out the feverish illnesses of childhood with antibiotics. The ego works through warmth and to take a new look at life you need to warm this inner spirit and get things moving. Iscador stimulates the thymus and raises the temperature, increasing white cells and antibodies. It is not claimed as a cure, rather as a contribution, a protector. It is often used before surgery, helping to encapsulate the tumour, making it easier to remove.

At Park Attwood – a beautiful house on an ancient ley line site in Worcestershire, set in seven acres of wooded parkland – a team of anthroposophists runs Britain's only residential clinic, where patients pay according to their ability and doctors are paid according to their need. It is a unique medical commune where practical duties, down to washing up, are shared by the doctors and nurses who believe that time shared with patients is a part of their therapy. Through learning to fuse paints on paper, in the unique Steiner way, cancer patients are loosened up and increase their capacity to express what is surging around inside. Fluidity is always the keynote of their approach: there is never a rigid, dogmatic attitude that 'this is automatically wrong'.

Food is organic and biodynamic, tending towards vegetarian but not rigidly so – there's no point in being rigid if someone is desperately ill. 'If someone has had a rubbishy diet and has the will to change an ingrained habit, that represents an enormous step – the ego taking hold and reshaping life.' Everywhere, the stress is on personal identity – rooms are bright and flower-filled, there is live music in the drawing room. Most of the patients at Park Attwood are not anthroposophists and are there following cancer surgery.

Homoeopathy

Homoeopathy is a system of medicine rather than a therapy, which uses herbs and minerals and is 'By Appointment' to the royal family. Queen Mary and King George VI were both devotees. Our Queen takes 'a battered black box full of medicines many chemists have never heard of . . . she uses arsenic for sneezing or an upset stomach, onion for a runny nose and anemone when someone is down in the dumps', according to James Whitaker, writing in the *Daily Star* in 1980.

The principle underlying homoeopathy is the reverse of that in allopathic or orthodox medicine. It is that the symptoms of any illness are produced by the defence mechanisms of the body fighting to ward off illness. Far from suppressing those symptoms, they should be given a helping hand. The homoeopath sees the introduction of drugs as rather like kicking a television set that is not working properly, whereas he prefers to track the disturbance to its root.

This is done on the basis that 'like cures like' – an idea going back to Hippocrates and Paracelsus. Thomas Sydenham, 17th century father of British medicine, had recommended that symptoms were seen as signs that disorder was being attacked by the patient's body. This idea was developed by Samuel Hahnemann in Germany 200 years ago. His studies of the effects of quinine, which had been used for centuries by South American Indians to treat malaria, led him to realise that the symptoms of malaria were not those of the disease but of the body's resistance to it.

Meanwhile, in Britain, Dr Edward Jenner was working on smallpox vaccines. Jenner became world famous and accepted by orthodox doctors, whereas Hahnemann pursued his researches one step further and so incurred the hostility of the profession and put homoeopathy entirely out of favour — where it has stayed. His theory, which rather unfairly made homoeopathy the whipping boy, was that the potency of a homoeopathic remedy did not depend on its strength but on its weakness. The more diluted, the greater the effect. It was utterly contrary to scientific sense, yet it worked.

Since homoeopaths were not allowed to practise (like anthroposophists) unless they had taken a full medical training and since during that training they were talked out of the feasibility of dilutions, the numbers of practising homoeopaths began eventually to diminish. In the fifties, when antibiotics and penicillin appeared and were successful, there seemed little hope for homoeopathy despite its inclusion in the newly created NHS.

But fashions change. Today, there is a certain disenchantment with the wonder drugs and a growing interest in a principle which has survived against heavy odds. One of its main assets is that there are no side effects with homoeopathic remedies.

There are NHS homoeopathic centres treating cancer in London, Liverpool, Glasgow, Bristol and Tunbridge Wells. There is a long waiting list and, whilst patients may continue to take any other drugs being prescribed if they wish, most people embarking on the homoeopathic path prefer to do so in a wholehearted and committed way. They are confident that the method works as well as any other and causes less distress en route.

Homoeopathic training is recognised by the state-controlled Faculty of Homoeopathy. The British Homoeopathic Association holds a list of medically qualified homoeopaths. Non-medically qualified practitioners are listed with the Society of Homoeopaths (see also Useful Addresses).

The Gerson Therapy

This is one of the toughest of all anti-cancer regimes, practical only for the most determined and self-motivated, for the natural fighters or those whose families are able to support them totally. It is not for the faint of heart or light of purse – for it is not recognised by the NHS or private insurance. You are on your own. It claims no miracle cure but its success rate is impressive.

Dr Max Gerson died in 1959, at a time before the alternative medicine movement had found a voice. His work has continued and is gaining further recognition. He was the pioneer of most nutritionally based therapies.

The Gerson Theory can be summed up as follows: cancer is not a specific, localised disease but a general chronic, degenerative one. Therefore, it is useless to remove tumours or try to eradicate other symptoms. They will only recur in a different location. Moreover, cancer is not so much a disease as a symptom: the symptom of a sick body system damaged over a long period of time.

In order to heal the body, it must be de-toxified and then activated with ionised minerals and naturally, organically grown food, so that the vital organs can function again. In practice, this means a strict vegan diet, coffee enemas, medication and a large intake of freshly made juices. It means a 24-hour-a-day effort to the exclusion of all else.

Beata Bishop is a writer who has described her personal experience of the Gerson therapy in *A Time to Heal*. She is adamant: 'It can be done – at home, in your own kitchen, with some help.'

> I should have died of malignant melanoma, one of the fastest spreading cancers, around June 1981. Today, I am healthy in the full sense of the word; not just not ill, but enjoying great well being and energy. When my secondary cancer was diagnosed in 1980 I was suffering from diabetes, osteoarthritis, frequent knock-out migraines and chronic dental abscesses. All those ailments have vanished. A large part of my right leg, mutilated by cancer surgery, has grown back. Doctors assure me that such regeneration is impossible, except that I happen to walk about on that impossibility every day of my life.

My journey from life-threatening disease to health was not a free trip. It cost me 18 months of close confinement on a tough, monotonous therapy that consumed most of my time and energy. It cost me my job and a great deal of money. It destroyed my lifestyle and forced me into an earthy, body-centred existence, a world away from my former mode of being that had been airy, colourful and focused on things of the mind. The journey also demolished my long-held self-image and through a series of inner upheavals forced me to take a fresh look at myself and acknowledge my shadow.

Beata first took the wholehearted, expensive step of travelling to La Gloria Hospital, the Gerson Clinic in Mexico, set amidst the 'deadly aridity' of borderland dust and disorder. No hibiscus and whitewashed houses here, just the worst excesses of twentieth-century American tattiness. The clinic grounds were luxuriant with cactus and palm trees but Beata's room was, she says, like a drab hotel room, 'refreshingly un-hospital like'.

Her book tells in graphic detail the physical and emotional obstacle race of the Gerson regime – 'a kind of desert crossing, a long slow trek through the wilderness . . . but blessed with a sprinkling of oases that grew brighter as time went on'.

Beata underwent the first two months of her course under the watchful eye of experts in Mexico, the next 16 months at home. She says:

Although my life was saved by the Gerson therapy, I do not claim it is the only alternative cancer treatment that works, only that it has the longest and best track record. Besides, most other unorthodox therapies are based on the Gerson diet. It is true that the intensive therapy is demanding, hard and boring, with a correspondingly high drop out rate . . . If anyone ever produces an easier and faster version that works just as well, I shall be the first to cheer loudly.

It is also true that the therapy is no panacea and carries no guarantee of a cure. No therapy does. What matters is that it views health and disease from a fresh, revolutionary angle which is still waiting to be discovered and understood by orthodox medicine.

In Britain there are a few physicians willing and able to supervise patients on the Gerson therapy. There is also a small network of lay helpers. Further information and advice is available from Ms Margaret Straus, Dr Gerson's granddaughter (see Useful Addresses).

The Issels Clinic – the Fever Folk

The Ringbergklinic is folded between mountain and lake in an especially beautiful part of West Germany at Bad Weissee. It was established by Dr Josef Issels in the early sixties, and its well-equipped, bathroom-en-suite, rooms have picture post-card views of the mountains. Josef Issels is one of Penny Brohn's 'Giants', described in her book *Gentle Giants*.

> Eventually we were led through treatment rooms mercifully free of the sad, ghost-like patients, to a white-tiled, white-walled, white-floored examination room. All glittering chrome and bright lights. We sat dazzled and blinking. David [her husband] looked even worse in this light. I told him to watch out or they'd be after him too and we both burst out laughing as Issels came in. . . . To say he 'came' into the room is not strictly accurate. He is a man who makes entrances and exits. He doesn't talk either, he makes utterances and statements, and he doesn't go in for 'soft-soap'.

The main thrust of the Issels approach is immunology, and although he uses radiotherapy and some cytotoxic drugs, his concern is to reawaken the body's own mechanisms for repelling disease. It is an endurance test at times more distressing than the disease itself. His particular bee is exercise . . . brisk walks up mountains on oxygenating jaunts. Like the anthroposophists, Dr Issels believes in raising the cancer patient's body temperature, through 'fever days'. Penny has described the misery of this time.

> Once a week we had to skip breakfast and started the day with an intravenous injection of B-coli virus. This had the double bonus effect of inducing a massive immune response in the body, stimulating a huge production of white cells and, at the same time, ensuring a significant rise in body temperature. The net effect of this was bad news for the cancer cells and none too terrific for the rest of you. I remember the fever days as a blur of pain, nausea, sickness and distress.

In the middle of one of these sessions, Dr Issels himself turned up. 'Get up. You must go out and walk. People die in bed – you must get up.' When she resisted, he snapped 'Do what you like. You are the one with cancer, not me.' 'I was shattered', she says, 'I dragged myself out for a walk. He was right.'

> Hour after hour I walked, through the woods and along the paths, sometimes taking a bus to explore a new place, sometimes braving

the terrors of the cable-car just for the thrill of flinging my arms out across the valley in a greeting to the unbelievable, distant, snow-capped peaks. I did a lot of arm-flinging and leaf-kicking and skipping over pavement cracks because I was making the most of being alone.

There is a world of difference between being alone and being lonely, just as there is between having cancer and being had by it. I kept telling myself that although I had cancer it hadn't got me, and thus, by taking some responsibility for having it, I felt I had some control over it as well. I tried a similar trick with being lonely. Of course there were days when I ached with longing for some real human contact, but at other times I embraced firmly the whole notion of being alone and cut off, and found it had some pleasing and satisfying side benefits.

It seemed as though I had never been alone before. Looking back through the perspective of my life I saw myself as having passed from a childhood – which had consisted largely of an earnest effort to please or achieve in the constant milling presence of parents or peers – almost without a break into young motherhood and the demands of three children born in the space of three years. Despite the pain of being parted from them there was a liberating joy in being with myself. I talked to myself a lot. Loudly. More than once I heard the approaching conversations of other walkers fade into embarrassed silence as they came towards me, passing this curious, mad Englishwoman with stiff nods and a murmured '*Guten tag*'. I didn't care a bit. I had no reputation here to worry about, no status to concern me. For the first time in years I allowed myself not to care what 'other people' thought, and it was strangely releasing.

Penny Brohn got better. She returned to Britain and co-founded the Bristol Clinic. Then, nearly four years later, she was threatened with a second tumour, and turned to Dr Ernesto Contreras.

The Contreras Clinic

This, like the Gerson clinic, is over the border, down Mexico way – another fugitive from the hard-line American drug companies. Penny Brohn went to Dr Contreras on the grounds that he might add to the knowledge she had gained from Josef Issels. The Clinico del Mar is an extremely beautiful, prosperous-looking place in the shadow of the grinding poverty of Mexican peasants. It costs at least £1,000 a week to be there.

Of all the clinics, Dr Contreras' combines the most therapies. He plays music personally to his patients on his guitar, he uses art and creates an atmosphere of peace and calm which is in itself healing. A few miles away he has built a hospital where chemotherapy, radiotherapy and surgery are also available for those who need them. Additionally, he has a team of nutritionists and psychologists, though his approach to diet is more relaxed than that of either Issels or Gerson. It is based on a belief that most people, if pushed too hard, will give up. So, although he proposes basically the same routine he allows for lapses. All this is glued together by a strong and deeply questing exploration of self and personality, backed, for those who want it, by religious experience. 'Most people are looking for someone to do a miracle – you must do the miracle yourself', he says.

The Contreras approach is understood and interpreted – rather less expensively – in Britain. The Bristol Centre and many others will supply information and help.

Dr William Kelley

Dr Kelley is an American with an impressive pedigree in orthodontics, chemistry, physiology, biology, education and a background of nutrition. His critics claim his methods are over-commercial. They are certainly expensive and have a touch of the evangelistic zeal that is a turn-off for the British, but what he is saying is sound. They are based on the same underlying principles as Gerson and Issels with some additional specialities.

Dr Kelley believes that cancer is an enzyme deficiency disease and that each individual requires individual treatment. To this end, he has devised a form comprising a 3,000 word questionnaire which costs £180 and, when filled in (an eight hour task!) is sent with urine and blood samples to the central computer in Dallas, Texas.

> The computer determines a design pattern or blueprint of a particular patient, diagnoses problems and gives suggested lines of action. Most people think that if you eat a balanced diet and take vitamins you will be healthy. It isn't as simple as that. You can eat the best organic foods and take all the vitamins in the world, but if your diet doesn't match your metabolism you are wasting your time and money.

Vitamin C can be a miracle cure for some, have no effect for others. Some people actually need meat. The Kelley Metabolic Typing Chart is a way of assessing your needs, and is a way of organising a lifestyle to suit your own nutritional requirements. Cancer patients, he says, need a fairly formidable daily intake of nutritional supplements which can be recommended by computer.

The Bournemouth Centre of Complementary Medicine is the chief exponent of Dr Kelley's method in Britain. This is a small residential clinic which aims to help patients follow whichever method they feel personally happy with.

Success Rates

An on-the-spot study of the Gerson, Contreras and Kelley methods by Dr Alec Forbes, a founder member of the Bristol Centre, and Tony Neate, now Chairman of New Approaches to Cancer, reported that their results appeared to have approximately the same success provided their regimes were thoroughly carried out:

Previously untreated cases of cancer with no detectable secondary spread	80–90 per cent became well and continued so on a mild maintenance regime
People failing on orthodox medical treatment with secondary spread	About 40–50 per cent became well and continued so on a mild maintenance regime
People previously treated by orthodox medical treatment and considered terminal	5–15 per cent became well and continued so on a mild maintenance regime

'If these claims are correct,' they said, 'they are better than orthodox medical treatment which gives a 50 per cent survival rate at 5 years for the first category and assures a practically 100 per cent failure rate for the second and third categories.'

Herbalism

There is nothing universally bad about chemotherapy or universally good about herbs. Let us be thankful for the choice.

From 'The Holistic Herbal', by David Hoffmann

Herbalism is an art and a science. Its prestige has been maligned and its use linked with magic and folklore. Herbs can be found free in the fields or ready prepared in certain health stores and chemists, but the qualified medical herbalist has undertaken a four-year course and has a professional knowledge of the role of herbs as an integral part of holistic medicine. Herbalism is not claimed as a guaranteed cure for cancer but a good herbalist, working alongside a GP or even a hospital consultant, can achieve spectacular results, even on tumours. Many of today's miracle drugs used in hospitals are based on herbs. For example, the Madagascan periwinkle is the source of drugs used in the treatment of leukaemia.

But the pure herbalist will claim this approach to specific cancers to be wrong – that no one herb should be used as an antidote to any one cancer. The treatment must be seen as a whole and cancer itself as a systemic disease of disorganisation, and that the correct herbs can be an invaluable aid to regaining control of the body. Such a transformation, say herbalists, is the only effective treatment.

The herbs most effective in healing tumours are Alteratives and Anti-neoplastics. Alterative herbs cleanse and normalise, and those that work through the liver are particularly good at helping the detoxification process: burdock, blue flag, yellow dock. The kidneys' eliminative function is helped by cleavers, also known as goosegrass, and dandelion. Those that have a tonic and cleansing action on the lymphatic system are especially important: cleavers, echinacea and poke root. The Anti-neoplastics are those which block the new growth, or neoplasm, which help to reassert order and structured organisation over the affected tissue.

The herbalist shares the view of most other alternative practitioners that cancer above all other diseases necessitates a holistic view of life. From this point of view, attitudes to diet and to the psychological causes of cancer are much the same. But David Hoffmann says 'We should remember that through aiding an organ with supportive and sustaining remedies, a renewal and release of vital energy will move the affected part of the body to cure itself of cancer.' As explained throughout his book, *The Holistic Herbal*, healing comes from the being's own life force and herbs can only facilitate this.

There are about 160 registered medical herbalists in Britain. Their register is available from the National Institute of Medical Herbalists (see Useful Addresses).

Bach Flowers

The 38 wild flower remedies which are still being prepared according to the original 1920 formulas of Dr Edward Bach are, he said 'absolutely benign in their action. They can never produce an unpleasant reaction under any condition and they can be safely prescribed and used by anyone.'

Trained as a pathologist and bacteriologist, Dr Bach switched to homoeopathy before the First World War. He came to believe that illness should be treated on the basis of individual personality and treatment aimed to counter the negative emotions which he believed caused illness. His colleague Norah Weeks says 'Throughout his years of medical practice he had been seeking for scientific proofs using his intellect, but a change came about. He became extremely sensitive to his intuitive faculty, for he found that by holding his hand over a flowering plant he would experience in himself the properties of the plant.' In other words, if he were worried, holding his hand over plants enabled him to find which would be appropriate to treat worry and its symptoms.

The remedies are available today in many health shops and there are practitioners nationwide. It is not unusual to find a holistic practitioner using Bach flowers in conjunction with other treatments. The Bach Centre at Wallingford near Oxford will supply them on request with their Handbook of Bach Flower Remedies. Bach flowers are suggested for people with an underlying emotional problem which may relate to physical symptoms: Fear . . . Rock Rose, Mimulus, Cherry Plum, Aspen, Red Chestnut; Despondency . . . Larch, Pine, Elm, Sweet Chestnut, Star of Bethlehem.

Help from: The Dr Edward Bach Centre (see Useful Addresses).

Meditation, Visualisation and Healing

A block of iron, symbolically lit from above by a single shaft of light is the centre of the Meditation Room at the United Nations in New York. It was designed by Dag Hamarskold as a centre of quiet peace where anyone, regardless of religious belief, may go for quiet communion with whatever spiritual power they recognise.

> After relaxing the body and centring the mind
> Enter the Meditation Room in thought and stand for a moment in its silence.
> Imagine it as a central point of the councils of the world.
> Visualise the room, with its symbolic altar in the centre and the shaft of light streaming steadily down upon it from on high.
> See this light reaching out to illumine the minds of each single member of the Assembly, and each one working in a place of responsibility.
> Hold this thought: see the light kindling in them forces of goodwill and light; send them your goodwill and light, asking that wisdom and compassion may illumine them in their work.
> Visualise light and goodwill radiating out from this place, reaching every country, people, place of conflict, crisis, suffering and need. *See* the difficulties resolving, the suffering lightening, the need being met, the conflict dying away, and hold this in the mind.
> Say aloud the following invocation, or any other that you prefer:
> May the Forces of Light bring Illumination to mankind.
> May the Spirit of Peace be spread abroad.
> May the Law of Harmony prevail.
> May men of goodwill everywhere meet in a spirit of cooperation.
> So let it be, and help us to do our part.
>
> *From 'The Silent Path' by Michael Eastcott*

Meditation is not the hobby of hippies, maharishis or Beatles. It is not a pagan ritual nor does it demand the wearing of saffron robes or nothing at all. It has, in fact, been an integral part of all the world's great religions and is equally valuable to the agnostic. The experienced practitioner can meditate on a tube or bus at will. Sadly, its reputation *has* been devalued by commercial bandwaggons. It can take a lot of time . . . but, remember, before you judge the idea as 'cranky' — there are strange doctors too!

Dr Ian Pearce is a family doctor whose work in the field of

cancer is greatly respected. He sees disease as a product of man's intransigence and that its healing will only come about by the restoration of wholeness and integration with the total environment. One way is through meditation and the work of the much-maligned healers.

In his thoughtful, kindly book, *The Gate of Healing* (which is best read before you are ill to extract full benefit) he says

> The great tragedy of the present time is that conventional medicine is so convinced of the rightness of its approach that it is not until this has been shown to have failed that patients start to look for additional help. By this time, it is often too late and the immune system and the general life forces of the body have been so damaged by the side effects of the normal therapy they no longer have the capacity to overcome the disease. Where meditation and diet are introduced from the outset before going for surgery the results are spectacular: operations proceed smoothly, post-operative healing is rapid and with minimal pain, and convalescence is speedy. Such patients are almost invariably 'star' patients in their wards, an example and an inspiration to others.

On a simple level, meditation can be more refreshing and restoring than deep sleep. Dr Pearce himself had been on hypnotics and anti-depressant drugs for some years following the death of his daughter. He was taught meditation by Dr Vincent Snell, an orthopaedic surgeon, who became leader of the Transcendental Meditation Movement in the UK. Six weeks later he was clear of all drugs – for ever.

There are many forms of meditation: 'a private and personal thing', a state which is neither dreaming nor sleeping nor waking, it is 'the fourth state'.

During meditation, all the body's responses to stress are put into reverse. The relaxation response was first described by Walter Hess in 1957: decrease in oxygen consumption, decrease in carbon monoxide elimination, reduction in heart rate, respiratory rate, blood pressure, blood lactate, muscle tone, blood cortisone levels, coupled with increase in circulation in the internal organs, rise in skin temperature of the fingers, increase in basal skin resistance, increase in alpha brain waves and the appearance of theta waves.

The cells of the brain are in a constant state of electrical activity, as was first discovered in 1875 by Richard Caton. Brain waves are minute alternating currents produced by this activity. The brain is divided into two sections – the left dealing with intellectual messages, the right abstract, holistic and artistic. That they are independent and literally the left does not know what the right is doing, is shown by the fact that they are not in any way synchronised.

During meditation, the level of activity, which varies according to the individual, progresses until the two sides become synchronous. Brain waves have been grouped into four now generally accepted groups. Of these, the alpha rhythm denotes 'an empty mind rather than a relaxed one, a mindless state rather than a passive one' (researcher Maxwell Cade). Described as a state of 'listening out', it is reduced by anxiety or mental concentration. The theta rhythm appears as consciousness moves towards drowsiness. 'In meditation', says Maxwell Cade, 'theta rhythm has been associated with alpha when it appears to be connected with access to unconscious material and creative inspiration. Individuals learn a profound sense of trust in their own inner experience and ways to allow their unique creativity to unfold.'

The first steps towards meditation are simple relaxation . . . and visualisation, in themselves valuable life lessons. The ingredients, according to Dr Herbert Benson of Harvard, are:

- A quiet, non-stimulating environment. Subdued lighting and silence are essential, especially for the beginner.
- A comfortable sitting position. Reduced muscle tone.
- A verbal or visual device to shift the mind towards internal imagining (a chanted word, a candle).
- A passive attitude. Don't worry if your mind wanders – let it, but be aware of what is happening.

Dr Ainslie Mears of Australia uses an adaptation of this technique:

Sit upright. Feet flat on the floor. Slide the left, and then the right, foot backwards and forwards until it feels neither back nor forwards. Hands hanging limply by the side of the chair. Sway the trunk backwards and forwards until it reaches a balance between the two. Repeat with the head and neck. Rest hands and forearms palms down on the thighs. Eyes are shut but behind closed lids are looking upwards towards the centre of the forehead. Then play either a tape (these can be bought in many health shops) or, if relaxing in a group, it's important that the leader's voice should not intrude but feel as though it is coming from within.

From this state of relaxation, a group instructor can move on into an exploration of the senses, an experience which must be all-absorbing and felt.

> You are standing within a garden on a summer's evening . . . It has been hot, and now, as the sun begins to sink, the trees, which give shelter to the garden, commence to cast long shadows across the lawns . . . Before you stretches a velvet green lawn, bordered by flowers, tall spikes of blue delphinium, lupins in red and yellow and blue, golden marigolds, against a backdrop of crimson roses and fragrant honeysuckle. You can hear the hum of the bees as they suck the nectar from the flowers . . . Above your head a gentle breeze rustles the leaves in the trees. . . .
>
> *Dr Ian Pearce, 'The Gate of Healing'*

If that is relaxation, what is meditation? It is a step further on, and it must be taught by an experienced teacher. In the wrong hands it can be dangerous. Krishnamurti the Indian sage once wrote 'Meditation is freedom from thought.' It serves to integrate our different levels of being. There are many ways of doing it but all involve two basic methods: focusing attention on an object of meditation such as a sound, or the breath, or a symbol, and opening up an attention to external and internal stimuli. It is the art of mind control and it is as relevant in the office as in the kitchen. In this state, the body enters a condition in which it becomes susceptible to the healing suggestions which the mind will presently make to it.

Most people know either of Zen meditation or transcendental meditation, but there are others — more movement-based such as Tai Chi, Karate and Sufi dancing. To discover the best method for you, you cannot do better than join an established group.

Most important, once learned, is to realise that meditation must become a part of the pattern of everyday life — a ritual that is as natural as brushing teeth. Meditation demands more dedication and discipline than relaxation. It requires a corner that is regularly 'special' and apart, and an atmosphere of reverence created by a particular picture, maybe some books, a candle, a joss stick. It is, if you like, the do-it-yourself version of a shrine. It requires time: a regular hour and a fixed time, best of all being dawn before the day intrudes, or sunset when the world is changing gear. A quarter of an hour may be enough.

Indian philosophy says that man is like a charioteer, whose job is to control the emotions and the intellect – the winged horses of the soul which, with the body, take the chariot forward. The chariot is life. The task of the charioteer – or 'I' – is to control the horses through reins – or thoughts – by which 'I' communicates with the soul. So 'I' is seen standing above the body, the emotions and the intellect, with a clear view of the road ahead controlling the journey.

Try this exercise devised by Roberto Assagioli, founder of Psychosynthesis:

Exercise in Dis-identification and recognition of the self
Sit quietly; systematically relax the body and close the eyes; slightly slow the breathing, starting by prolonging the outbreaths to a count of four or five in seconds; pause for a second before breathing in over a similar period. Keep this going for two or three minutes, until you have got a gentle rhythm going which can be maintained without concentration or effort.

Say slowly and with sincerity: if preferred, this can be recorded on tape, when working alone.

1 *I have a body*, but *I am not my body*. With my body I relate to the world around me, but *I am not* my body. My body may be tired or rested, sick or well, wakeful or sleeping, but it is only a house in which I dwell and through which I work and express myself. *I have a body* but *I am not my body*.

2 *I have* emotions, but *I am not* my emotions. They are for ever fluctuating and changing. I may feel happiness or sadness, joy or despair, anger or peace. I can watch and judge my emotions: I can control them to a limited degree. With my emotions I relate to those in the world around me, but *they are not* myself. *I have* emotions, but *I am not* my emotions.

I also have desires, likes and dislikes. They are too fluctuating and changeable, but *they are not* myself. *I have* emotions, but *they are not myself*.

3 *I have* a mind, but *I am not* my mind. I can control and direct my mind. It is unruly, but it is teachable. It is an organ of consciousness both of the world within and of the world without, but *it is not myself. I have* a mind, but *I am not my* mind.

4 I am neither my body, my emotions nor my mind. *I am a centre of pure self-consciousness. I am a centre of will*, able to master and control my body, my emotions and my mind. *I am a centre of light, the pure, unchanging self that lives within.*

Healing

> There are no miracles only ignorance.
>
> *Pythagoras*

If there is more to meditation than saffron robes and joss sticks, there is more to healing than witchcraft and miracles. At its worst, healing is quackery practised by self-important, intense amateurs, and, at its best, can appear, almost miraculously, to move mountains. But healing does not fit into any accepted medical pattern and is, therefore, dismissed by the majority of doctors, though the BMA have been running controlled trials. They say that the so-called miracle cures can be accounted for in one of three ways:

1   They would have occurred anyway.
2   The placebo effect – what the mind expected was caused to happen – autosuggestion. This is often what happens in the hysterical reaction to mass faith healing and it seldom lasts.
3   The condition did not exist in the first place.

The healers themselves are convinced that energy channelled through the hands can be activated by the mind of one person and so trigger off changes in another. Healers do not generally call themselves faith healers. They believe that healing can happen with or without faith; some see it as a manifestation of God's power, others as a paranormal, natural occurrence. Either way, it is an ancient phenomenon known to mankind of all religions and all levels.

The tribal witch-doctor or medicine man was a combined priest, holy man and healer. He achieved his magic through trances and ritualised dance. Gradually, the art of healing was displaced by the belief that illness was a sign of God's wrath and there wasn't much point in contradicting Him. Christianity changed that. Jesus said 'Preach the gospel, heal the sick' and the New Testament is a chronicle of almost every possible kind of healing.

Healing became woven into Christian practice. But gradually as the medieval fear of witchcraft arose, the practice of spiritual healing became linked with mumbo jumbo, trances and hysteria . . . and was exorcised. All that was left was a shadowy, superficial ritual. In the thirteenth century, priests were forbidden to practise medicine and spiritual healers were outlawed. Church and medicine separated for ever. This is the legacy of suspicion that survives today. But spiritual healing is not the prerogative of the Christian church and there are many secular forms being practised in the eighties.

Christian Science Founded at the end of the 19th century by Mary Baker Eddy, holds that physical ills, including cancer, can be tackled by faith and prayer.

Spiritualism Also a Victorian phenomenon, whose followers included Sir Arthur Conan Doyle. Spiritualist healers believe they can cure the sick by communication with 'the other side', that they themselves are the medium by which healing works. Spiritualist churches sprang up around the country and challenged the staid attitudes of the Established Church. Gradually, many denominations revived varying forms of healing. Spiritualists believe that healing is available to non-believers.

Harry Edwards was the Spiritualist missionary who awoke the great tide of public interest in the fifties and who founded the National Federation of Spiritual Healers. His reputation as a curer of cancer, TB and arthritis seems well founded.

In 1977, the year after his death, the then General Medical Council wrote to the NFSH and climbed down, after years of hostility. Doctors were at last to be allowed to associate with spiritual healers and not be struck off the register. 'The President can see no reason why a doctor should not, if he considers that it would be helpful to one of his patients, either suggest or agree to a patient seeking assistance from a member of your Federation, provided the doctor himself continued to give and to remain responsible for whatever medical treatment he considered necessary for the patient.' It was a truce.

Today Spiritualism no longer plays a dominant role and the work of most healing organisations is under the auspices of the Confederation of Healing Organisations. They have encouraged the setting up of standards, educational programmes and tests in conjunction with orthodox medical authorities.

Laying on of hands Many churches and religious organisations now offer this service as therapy, either in a church, at home or in hospital.

Charismatic healing 'Speaking in tongues', is practised by charismatic Christians and is based on St Luke's 'there appeared unto them cloven tongues like of as fire and it sat upon each of them.' It is a response to a basic urge for free expression and open release of spiritual forces – and so healing powers.

Hand healing is not the same as the Christian laying on of hands. It is more secular and detached . . . untouched by the divine. 'Stroking' as it was first called in the seventeenth century, involved passing the hands up and down the body, not necessarily touching, and smoothing the pain or hurt out, in much the same way as a schoolboy imparts magnetism to a steel by stroking it with a magnet. Many hand healers believe their power is a form of bio-electromagnetism which is present in all but active in some and can be developed by anyone.

Remember Leonid Brezhnev, forever at the point of death according to newspapers: he appeared, despite rumours of terminal illness, to be indestructible. His apparent improvement, according to reports, was due to a former waitress, the young Dzhuna Davitashvili, a healer who was being paid around £1,745 a session by leading Russian public figures.

Because healing has been grudgingly accepted by doctors, British healers are in demand worldwide. Probably best known is Matthew Manning, who has worked with doctors and scientists anxious to learn more of his powers. Cancer is one of the diseases he is often asked to treat. He makes no claims for miracles. He believes that 90 per cent of cases are triggered by an emotional trauma, usually divorce or bereavement, and that patients are committing mental suicide. Healing can only help to move them away from that state of mind towards a new love of life.

How to find a healer you can trust:

- If a healer does not request that you are also in the care of a doctor, he is probably a charlatan.
- If he promises cures, he is a quack.
- If he charges you large sums, beware.

But if a healer is to work, he may not have time to earn a living and a charge for his time is in order – especially when, like

Matthew Manning, your popularity demands a secretary and formidable expenses.

Help from the following, who are listed in Useful Addresses: Harry Edwards Healing Sanctuary; Matthew Manning Centre; National Federation of Spiritual Healers.

Help for non-believers Those with a religious faith believe and accept the power of prayer as a direct contact with God. Those who are fence-sitters may like to think of it in a rather different context – as a very personal way of letting go . . . unwinding . . . expressing thoughts. Talking to yourself can be a therapeutic exercise if you understand what you are doing. Cancer patients in need of spiritual rafts to cling to but who are wavering in their attitude to spiritual matters, who feel they can't manage on their own but don't believe in a listening God, may find the Humanist Association helpful. Humanism aims to establish a set of beliefs and moral ideals which are free from religious doctrine. It provides a framework for living which concentrates on 'the mental and moral improvement of the human race' as a worthy end in itself.

Help from: British Humanist Association (see Useful Addresses).

Bone Breathing Visualisation

The Chinese believe that the centre of your bones is responsible for the well-being of the body as a whole. This exercise in visualisation, together with the relaxation that goes with it, is being widely used for therapy for those with bone disorders. You will use your breath by imagining the breath entering up and through the bones as you breathe in, and as you breathe out it passes down and away through the same path.

The first thing is to get yourself into a comfortable position, either:

1 In the sitting position, in a comfortable upright chair, feet placed evenly on the floor, hands resting in the lap, spine straight, and the head resting comfortably, the top of the head in line with the ceiling.

(or) 2 Lying down on a comfortable mat, with the spine as straight as possible, arms to the side, with the palms uppermost, feet just a little way apart.

Begin to become aware of your breathing, slow the breath right down, getting it as slow and deep as you can. Feel the breath right down in to the bottom of the ribcage as you breathe in deep, slow, even breathing. Begin to feel the body relaxing as you just concentrate your mind on the breath as it comes in and out, relaxing and letting go.

Now imagine your body:

1   Imagine the breath coming in and up through the bones of the left foot, up the bones of the leg to the hip bone. Then as you breathe out, the breath returns the same way and out through the left foot. Repeat 7 times.

2   Then imagine the breath coming in and up through the bones of the right foot, up the leg and up to the hip and then, as you breathe out, the breath returns the same way and out through the right foot. Repeat 7 times.

3   Now breathe in through the bones of the left foot up the left leg, cross over through the pelvis and, as you breathe out, send the breath out and down the bones of the right leg, and out through the right foot. Breathe in and up the right foot and up through the leg, cross over the pelvis and down the left leg, and out through the left foot. Repeat 7 times.

4   Now breathe in and up through the bones of the left hand, up through the bones of the left arm to the shoulder, breathe out and return down and out the same way. Repeat 7 times.

5   Now breathe in and up through the bones of the right hand and up the right arm, to the shoulder, then breathe out and down the same way. Repeat 7 times.

6   Breathe in and take breath in through the left hand, up the left arm, across from the left shoulder to the right, then, breathing out, down the right arm and out through the bones of the right hand. Breathe in and up the right hand, up the right arm to the shoulder, across to the left shoulder, and breathe out down the left arm and out through the left hand. Repeat 7 times.

7   Breathing in, take the breath up the spine to the top, and then, as you breathe out, send the breath down the spine again and out through the base. Repeat 7 times.

8   Imagine the skull: take a breath in and up and over the head to the front, breathing out, take the breath through the skull and back. Repeat 7 times.

9   Now imagine the body as a whole. Take the breath in, up from both feet and up through all the bones in the body to the top of the head, breathing down and out through all the bones and out through the feet. Repeat 7 times.

It may be easier to visualise the breath in terms of a colour, or a light, or a feeling of warmth, whichever you find the easiest, and repeat the whole exercise as often as you like. It may seem a little difficult at first, but persevere and soon it will flow and you will receive great benefit.

Macrobiotics – the Seaweed People

Macrobiotics is a Japanese vegetarian diet based on eastern ethical beliefs and a very strict lifestyle. To achieve any kind of success it requires such a radical change from western methods that, for an already anxious, sick person, it can be too hard and therefore counter-productive. Alternatively, provided a patient is keen and has the full care and support of his family it may provide a disciplined incentive for fighting.

Macrobiotic principles were brought to the west in the fifties by Michio Kushi, renowned authority on eastern medicine. Diet, he said, should be based on a balance of yin and yang foods. The Japanese classification of yin and yang differs from the Chinese and anyone interested in macrobiotics should seek further explanation from the East-West Foundation in London. Each person has different yin and yang dietary needs, and the composition of all foods can be altered by their method of growing and preparation. Colour in diet is also extremely important.

According to the East-West Foundation publication *The Cancer Prevention Diet*, 'When cancer develops a greenish shade will often appear on the skin. The appearance of this colour represents a process of biological degeneration.'

Among the seven primary colours, red has the longest wavelength and is more yang. The opposite colours – purple, blue and green – have shorter wavelengths, are cooler and, therefore, more yin. Red is the colour of the more yang animal kingdom and is apparent in the colour of blood. On the other hand, vegetables, which are yin, are based on green chlorophyll. Eating represents the process whereby we transform green vegetables into red animal blood.

The more yin colours – purple and blue – appear in the sky and atmosphere, both of which are the more expanded yin components of the environment. The more yang colours – yellow, brown and orange – appear in the compacted world of minerals.

During the transformation of vegetable life into human blood and cells, waste products are eliminated through functions such as urination and bowel movements. These represent the in-between stages and, therefore, are yellow and brown colours which lie between the green and red in the spectrum.

Cancer is a reverse process in which body cells decompose and revert towards vegetable life. This is manifested in the appearance of a greenish tinge on a part of the body corresponding to the site of the disease.

Region where the greenish tinge might appear

Small intestine	Outside of little finger
Lung	Either or both cheeks
Stomach	Along the outside of both legs, especially below the knee
Bladder	Around either ankle or the outside of the leg
Liver	Around the top centre of the foot

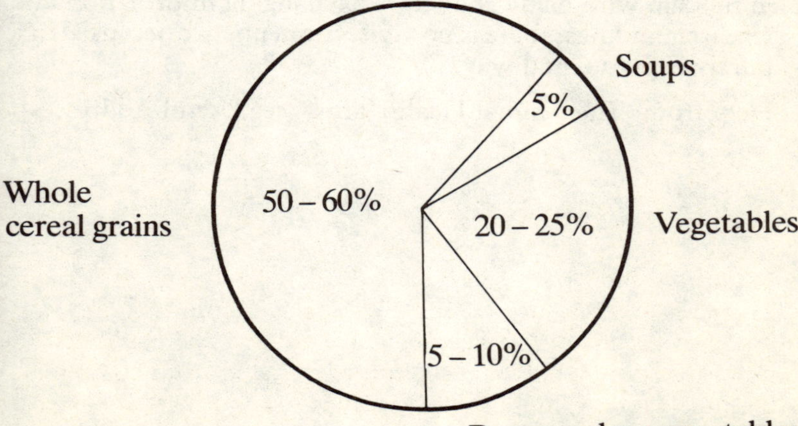

Some cancers can result from an excess of yin foods, others from an overdose of yang, whereas others arise from an excess of both extremes. To offset the development of cancer it is important to recover a balance in diet. The standard macrobiotic diet is shown in the diagram but the same dietary programme should not necessarily be adopted for every case and macrobiotics should not be followed without medical advice and consultation with a macrobiotic specialist.

Care for Pets with Cancer

Animals are known to have had cancer long before the appearance of man on earth. Today, more dogs than humans die of the disease annually; distressed pet owners often telephone the cancer help groups for advice about sick cats and dogs. As in humans, early treatment and diagnosis can help the chance of survival.

The Animal Health Centre at Newmarket in Suffolk is the only charitable institution in Great Britain investigating full time the diagnosis, care and prevention of animal diseases, especially cancer, and caring for them in its hospital. The Oncology Unit is being fitted with all the latest equipment and a team of veterinary surgeons and medical staff are working to relieve pain and improve life for hundreds of pets. They work in tandem with medical doctors exchanging information and research findings; there is no vivisection, nor are pets used in a purely experimental way.

Help from: The Animal Health Trust (see Useful Addresses).

8
Children With Cancer

There is so much light as well as shade in the story of children with cancer. For despite the inescapable, indescribable agony tearing all parents, the desperate confusion and guilt that one so young can suffer, children themselves often see their situation differently. They are protected by their innocence; often too young to be burdened with pessimism or a fear of dying, they can be remarkably positive, even cheerful.

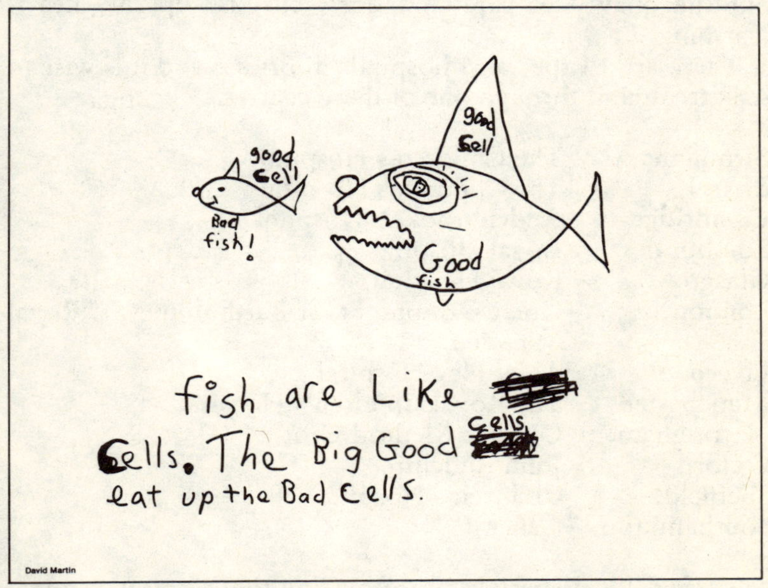

Of course, it is not always like that. There is pain; there may well be tears, but even so the children's ward can appear a disarmingly happy place. This places a terrible burden on any family, one which is not at all the same as caring for adults. The needs of healthy children change rapidly as they grow.

They are learning at a phenomenal rate and parents adapt to these changes, feeling their way, maybe making mistakes along the road. But once a child has cancer, natural parental confidence is shaken, guilt overshadows all and there is no longer time to make mistakes. As a result, the understandable urge is to spoil and protect the young invalid and so to set him or her apart, but it is an urge which any children's nurse will advise against. So parents have the double agony of continuing life as normally as possible: the training, the teaching, the loving, the discipline, knowing it may all be in vain.

Childhood cancers are rare, accounting for only 1 per cent of all cases, although they are second only to accidents as the most frequent cause of death in children aged three to fourteen. Their prognosis is improving all the time. Perhaps because they are uncommon, there is less widespread support for parents than for families looking after adults with cancer, but the quality of care that does exist is superbly heart-warming.

There are 14 specialist hospitals in Britain and it is wise to seek treatment through one of these centres.

Birmingham	The Children's Hospital
Bristol	The Children's Hospital
Cambridge	Addenbrooke's Hospital
Edinburgh	Royal Hospital
Glasgow	Royal Hospital
London	Great Ormond St, St Bartholomew's, Royal Marsden
Liverpool	Alder Hey Hospital
Manchester	The Royal Children's Hospital
Nottingham	Queen's Medical Centre
Oxford	John Radcliffe
Sheffield	Children's Hospital
Southampton	General

To find local specialist care outside the hospital is much more difficult for there is an acute shortage of trained children's nurses.

Perhaps it is helpful to see the story through the compassionate eyes of some of the few dedicated to caring for children with cancer.

Bernadette Cleary

Bernadette Cleary has devoted herself to the care of dying children at home. Bernadette, herself the youngest of a family of 15 who grew up in two rooms, is the mother of three young boys and former foster parent to another 56 over a period of seven years. For seven days a week, 52 weeks a year she is ready to pack her bags and travel from her Surrey home to ease the heartache of any family who needs her. She makes no charge and covers her costs by donations from well-wishers and, in between visits, charring and teaching. Ninety per cent of her work is on the breadline level or below, in places where there is appalling overcrowding and water running down the walls. Her wisdom and understanding of parents, patients and their siblings is probably unique, adapting equally to orthodox or holistic methods, to the religious or to the non-believer. She wears no uniform, is 'trained in nothing' and yet is greatly respected by all the doctors who have worked with her. Despite her own holistic beliefs, she would not dream of being a missionary for these methods. 'The secret of real help is to start where the family is – not where you would like them to be,' she says.

> I support the family in what they want for their child and at whatever level of caring they need. Sometimes, it is just more useful to go shopping than try to change a junk food diet. The art is not to judge, just to get on and do the job and to make dying more easy. It is so important to work with the entire family: parents get blown apart, to treat them all, especially the brothers and sisters who are so often neglected and suffer appallingly.

Her theme is always TLC – tender loving care. She is a fervent believer in the power of touch, especially in massage with aromatic oils and the gentle stroking of feet. 'I encourage holding and touching between all the family.' Pain she relieves with colour visualisations, colour breathing and relaxing pale blue baths, and special lighting that brings peace. Children are more open about cancer and often good at trying new techniques. They have less clutter in their minds and with such vivid imaginations find visualisation a natural idea. 'Tell them to breathe rose pink into the lungs, and they will understand and respond. They enjoy simple yoga, too', she says. At all times she encourages discussion and sharing of thoughts.

Her dream is the foundation of Rainbow House, a holistic hospice where others can be trained in the work she has pioneered. 'It will be a resting place for the entire family during a very difficult time. A home from home where people have time to listen, to share and to support. Where basic needs such as washing, ironing and cooking can recede, giving the family more time for themselves. We have many opportunities to learn when we bring a child into the world – pre-natal and ante-natal care – but there is a need for the same opportunities on the outward journey.'

Help from: Bernardette Cleary (see Useful Addresses).

The Centre for Attitudinal Healing

Gerry Jampolsky is an 'original' – an American psychiatrist whose methods have breathed fresh air into the claustrophobic world of terminal cancer.

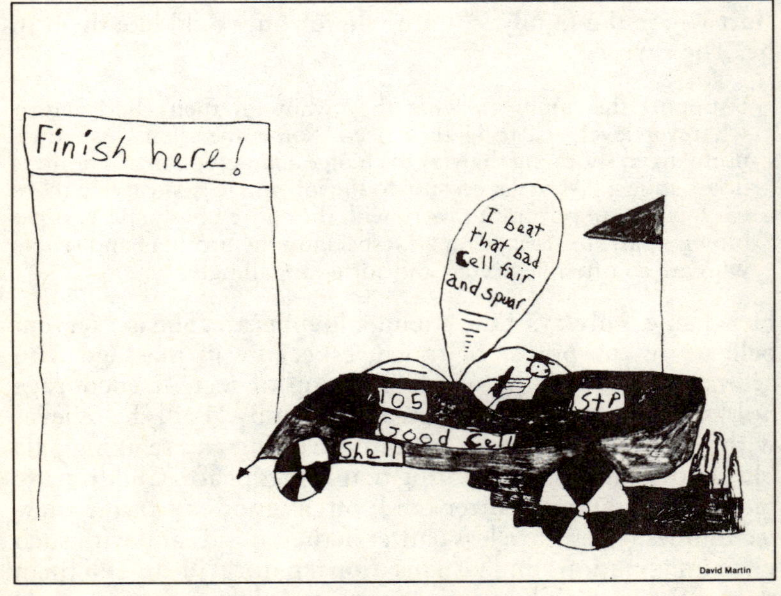

At a Centre for Attitudinal Healing you may find bald-headed children discussing chemotherapy and how to cope with the teasing of classmates, and parents learning to speak honestly about their anger and fear. Meditation, games and drawing are all part of the course. 'When adults and children work together to see life clearly from a sense of inner peace, attitudes shift. Healing can then begin from a spiritual level.'

'Sick children', he says, 'develop wisdom, peace and maturity.' He began to base his work upon that wisdom, and upon the writings of an American spiritual book *A Course in Miracles*, which provided a ladder to self-awareness and peace of mind. *A Course in Miracles* was a spiritual revelation to a Jewish atheist called Helen Schucman in 1970. It is transformational writing, claiming to awaken new attitudes at a deeply personal level.

This is no soft option. There are no platitudes at one of the Jampolsky Centres – no rose-coloured spectacles allowed. Children and their families are taught to face the truth about the illness and learn to express their real needs. A child can do this in a day whereas adults take much longer to uncover a lifetime's inhibitions. There are no miracle cures, no remission statistics, yet families leave feeling better and happier. There is no charge and all workers are voluntary.

Help from: Centre for Attitudinal Healing (see Useful Addresses).

The Children's Cancer Help Centre

The first centre established solely for the care of children with cancer and their families was opened in Lewisham, London in 1986. It is run by Suzanne Kruger, a children's nurse who cured herself of cancer, and Julia Collet, trained in psychosynthesis. The aim is to support a family in whatever choice of treatment they have chosen for their child, though help and advice are offered from a holistic point of view. Contributions are voluntary.

Families arrive at midday bringing lunch to share, though Julia and Suzanne provide salads and talk about nutrition and diet over the meal. Fathers are always encouraged to be there but very often are reluctant. After lunch, Suzanne takes the children off to paint and play, to have hand healing and learn meditation. 'We like the children to be apart from parents because the parents have their own work to do and, besides, children open up more on their own,' she says.

Very often Julia and Suzanne are asked to help after the death of a child – 'We never do anything unless we are asked. That's why we prefer families to approach us themselves in the first place rather than be referred although we then liaise with their GP. We want to be sure it is they, the parents, who want to try our approach.'

It is hoped that a second centre in the north of England may be open before long. In the meantime, the one at Lewisham is unique.

Help from: The Children's Cancer Help Centre (see Useful Addresses).

A Mother's Way

On Thursday, 18 June 1970, American journalist Mikie Sherman telephoned her doctor because her four and a half year old daughter, Elizabeth, was under par and had developed

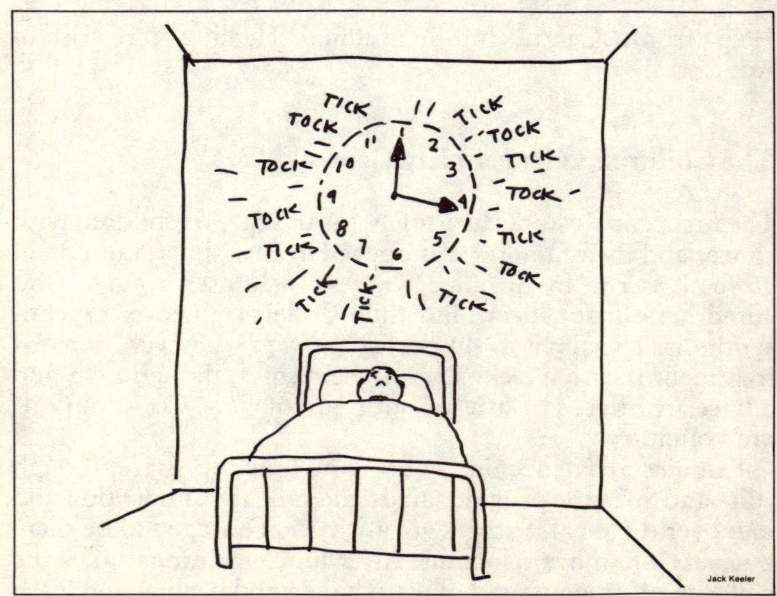

swollen neck glands. Within ten days she was told that the little girl had leukaemia. Two and a half years later, Elizabeth died 'my arm around her shoulder, her head on my breast'.

Mikie Sherman wrote a short, parent-to-parent account of those years in which she described some of her own reactions and feelings. They may help.

The leukaemic child has, at the least, undergone a period of hospitalisation and painful medical treatment. His concept of self – of bodily integrity, capabilities, energies, vulnerability – has been severely damaged, and will not immediately be repaired in remission. Relapses may succeed remissions, and the two may be separated by long grey periods when he is neither really sick nor really well. Subsidiary complications, infections and toxic drug reactions can occur. The parent attempts to deal with these bewildering and unpredictable changes out of a basic context of anxiety and fear, perhaps physical and financial strain. Little wonder that the world of both parent and child can become dominated by feelings of uncertainty, alienation, and loss of normalcy.

All will be reflected in the child's behaviour. Here again, as in the hospital, his basic stance may be one of either withdrawal or overt expression of hostility. Elizabeth, generally withdrawn in the hospital, became angry at home. She laboured, I felt, under a tremendous sense of frustration, frustration produced, I believe, by all those leukaemia related effects which made her feel different from other children – loss of hair and weight gain caused by drugs; frequent tiredness; weakness in her legs; recurring infections; weekly medical treatment. She resented terribly not being able to keep up, and, in living with her disabilities, her resentment took the form of anger.

Her anger manifested itself in many ways, and almost always at home, where she knew it would usually be accepted and understood. She became very possessive about some of her belongings – a chair in the kitchen, for instance – and would react violently if they were used by another person; she became very hostile toward anyone who would interrupt a private game or ritual of hers; she demanded the bulk of the time I spent at home and was very jealous of any persons who seemed to infringe on it.

These behaviour patterns were not continuously present, but they did persist well into a remission, surfaced occasionally during its course, and reappeared before a physically diagnosed relapse had occurred. When she was obviously ill, they were relatively easy to deal with, as I and other members of the family were able to make the needed special allowances. At other times it seemed almost impossible to cope with my own conflicts, as what had earlier figured as special treatment deserved by the sick seemed to become over-indulgence of an overly demanding child. Yet I could never handle her outbursts of temper as easily as I could those of a completely well child, primarily for two reasons – often I feared that she was becoming sick, in the slow, insidious way of leukaemia, and this feeling was reinforced by the fact that this sometimes subsequently proved to be the case; and always I was aware of the tremendous burden of frustration she carried.

Whether I was overly indulgent with Elizabeth I do not know; I still have no answer. I certainly wish I had at times been able to handle the situation better, for in meeting Elizabeth's needs, as I perceived them, my two older children were often perforce relegated to the back. Often I could not cope with Elizabeth's demands for my time or her angry reactions and at the same time provide for my older children the attention they needed and the protection their rights deserved when they became embroiled in a conflict with her. I wanted the older children both to treat her with special consideration and treat her 'normally'. They were of course confused, as were we all; yet there were times of rare understanding and helpfulness.

From 'The Leukaemic Child' by Mikie Sherman

Feeding the Child with Cancer

At the best of times, feeding children can be a bumpy ride; either they tackle meals with the voraciousness of a waste disposal unit or they are faddy pickers, happy on a diet of beefburgers and crisps. To force a child who is really ill, and feeling terrible, into new eating habits probably won't work and may not do much good. It depends greatly on just how ill they are, and if they are mature enough to cooperate.

The sensible cancer nutrition plan already laid out for adults applies as much to children, but it is sometimes better for youngsters, especially the terminally ill, to stick with the familiar rather than battle over something new. So don't worry too much about ice cream and jelly. Use your own common sense but, for instance, avoid fry-ups where possible. A little diplomacy – in restricting sweets from visitors and selecting fresh juices rather than over-coloured cordials – is wise but this is the best level of monitoring rather than a sudden slashing of all the goodies that make a really ill child's life bearable.

Amanda Brown

For 19-year-old Amanda Brown's family, the thrill of watching her jump a clear round in the local gymkhana was a miracle. Four years ago, at the age of 15, Amanda was 'within hours' of dying at the Royal Marsden Hospital, Sutton in Surrey. She'd been taken ill after feeling 'funny' at Wimbledon, and, though she had never been ill in her life, was found to have a massive number of leukaemic cells. The course of treatment prescribed – Berlin Protocol – was so horrendous that few adults have had it, fewer have been able to cope. It involves regular lumbar punctures, daily injections, bone marrow transplants (from the sternum or the ileac crest) and huge doses of chemotherapy and radiation.

Her Dad promised her the best horse he could buy if she recovered, and Amanda accepted the challenge.

'At first I thought I had glandular fever,' she says, 'but when they transferred me to a different hospital and I heard the ambulance driver say "Royal Marsden" I knew what was wrong. That was the worst moment in my life – I was really scared. They took me to the ward and I felt terrified, seeing all those people with bald heads. I remember crying then.

'I wanted to know what my chances were, and when the doctor said 70 per cent, I knew I had to get over it. I think I have a low pain threshold. I was pretty strong and although the treatment hurt at first I learned to relax and it seemed better. Once the treatment started I felt better anyway. I didn't really have time to think about dying. I knew the nurses could only do so much. The rest was up to me.'

Amanda's Mum stayed with her all the time, often leaving the hospital after she was asleep at midnight. Friends flooded her with nearly 500 cards; and gradually she improved. In 1984, Amanda was cleared and taken off drugs – though she still takes the vitamins which her parents feel helped greatly to give her strength.

She achieved her dream horse 'Killarney Kate' and is now working in the local chemist shop near Sutton, Surrey. 'I am an only child – and I think having cancer softened me – I was a bit spoilt and a bit of a handful at school. Being so ill makes you really appreciate life and makes you aware of what is important. I feel more relaxed and much more tolerant now, and much more aware of others. I haven't become a goody goody, but I try to be nicer than I was.'

Childhood Cancers

Leukaemia

Leukaemia is probably the best known of the childhood cancers. But although there are several types of leukaemia, only one – acute lymphocytic leukaemia – is common in children between the ages of two and seven and accounts for one third of cases. Symptoms are rather vague: tiredness, recurring infection, bruising or bleeding, enlarged lymph glands or spleen (situated on the left of the abdomen), bone pains.

The treatment is usually by chemotherapy, to which this particular cancer responds well so that there is now a good chance of complete cure. As with adults, the effects of chemotherapy are often hard to bear, especially as children are cruel to each other and the loss of hair can be a terrible trial at school. Leukaemic children are particularly prone to infection so that they must be protected to a degree. The first six months is the most difficult time when the child is undergoing intensive treatment. The magic word for all parents of a leukaemic child is 'remission' – this usually occurs after about one month of such treatment and can last for a varying amount of time – maybe a year, maybe five, maybe more. The longer the remission the less the chance of a relapse and after ten years this becomes unlikely. During remission, treatment is no longer necessary.

Lymphoma

The treatment of Hodgkin's disease and non-Hodgkin's lymphoma is not the same for children as for adults. The difference between Hodgkin's and other lymphomas is marked by the existence of an abnormal cell, the Reed-Steinberg cell, in the lymph nodes. The prognosis is good and improving, despite these being fast-growing tumours.

They are usually treated with a combination of radiotherapy and chemotherapy rather than surgery, though treatment will depend on the stage the disease has reached when diagnosed. Hodgkin's disease tends to appear in the late teens and is more common among boys. The symptoms are generally a swollen lymph gland, often in the neck, but unexplained fever, night sweats and weight loss are also pointers. Occasionally, itching occurs.

Non-Hodgkin's Lymphoma The symptoms are not the same as in Hodgkin's disease. They can be a tumour in the chest causing shortness of breath, bowel stoppages and other bowel or stomach problems, enlarged lymph nodes or glands and possibly enlargement of tonsils or adenoids. Treatment is complex and variable; side effects can be traumatic but are made bearable by the increasing hopes of success.

Fiona Burns

Fiona Burns is 21 – a student nurse at Manchester Royal Hospital working a heavy day and, like most girls of her age, 'burning the candle at both ends'.

When Fiona was 12 years old she was so weak and run down that she had no strength to feed her pet rabbit at the end of the garden. The bruise on her leg caused by a bang on a school peg didn't heal, but for six months the doctors could find nothing wrong.

Eventually, after operations, biopsies and bone marrow tests, the consultant told Mrs Burns they had found malignant cells and that Fiona had multiple myeloma – a cancer associated usually with old age. They said that chemotherapy was the treatment. They also said that Fiona would need regular treatment for the rest of her life. They gave no suggestion how long that could be. 'Her long, wavy fair hair was coming out, she was sick and I just kept asking myself "What am I doing to her?" ' recalls Mrs Burns.

Mr and Mrs Burns decided to try Fiona on the Gerson diet – an extremely strict vegetarian regime also involving daily coffee enemas (see pages 126–7). They explained to Fiona she was suffering from 'toxicity'. When her Mum offered 50p per enema, 20p for breakfast, 30p for lunch and also joined in the diet, she agreed to cooperate, even though, like any other teenager, she didn't think much of it all.

Within 6 months, Fiona was back at school. Her energy returned and has never flagged. Her mother returned the drugs – kept safely in a plastic bag – to a surprised but impressed consultant. Not till Fiona was 17 did her parents tell her what it was all about because she was smoking and going to parties.

Today, having worked on a cancer ward herself, she has a very personal understanding of what it means.

Bone Tumours

The symptoms are pain and swelling of the bone and restricted limb movement.

Chondrosarcoma This is a slow growing tumour of the bone and is treated usually by surgery. If the tumour is large, amputation may be necessary but usually the removal of the growth and surrounding bone is very successful.

Ewing's Sarcoma This occurs between the ages of five and sixteen and is more common amongst boys. Usually a biopsy is necessary as it is not easy to differentiate between a Ewing's sarcoma and other tumours. Treatment is very high doses of radiation and, because such doses may cause impaired movement, a programme of exercise is planned to keep the patient as mobile as possible. The high radiation dose also causes soreness and very often skin thickening. Because this is a fast-spreading tumour, chemotherapy is used as well to eradicate any hidden metastases. The cure rate is rising but this is still a particularly vicious form of cancer that requires a great deal of stamina from both patient and family.

Soft Tissue Sarcoma

These are rare tumours of the soft tissue — most common in the muscle. They are identified by swellings and usually treated by a combination of chemotherapy, radiotherapy and surgery. Horrific as the side effects of these methods may appear, children are remarkably resilient and cope, on the whole, better than adults, but the future will depend very much on the site of the original tumour.

Neuroblastoma These account for about one in ten cases of childhood cancer, mostly in children under two years old. The cure rate for these young patients is good unless widespread. But as the tumour grows from cells known as sympathetic nerves, which are widespread throughout the body, the tumour can arise in several places and tends to spread via the lymphatics. Symptoms are: prolonged jaundice after birth, swelling in the neck or abdomen, coughing, high blood pressure, weight loss, poor appetite and occasionally a protrusion of the eye. These tumours produce a substance called catecholamines which can be detected in urine. Treatment is, again, a combination of radiotherapy, surgery and chemo-therapy according to the staging of the disease and its location.

Wilms' Disease Wilms' tumour occurs more commonly in children with birth abnormalities, such as those in the urogenital system, absence of the iris in the eye or over-growth of half the body. Again, very young children respond well to treatment and generally surgery is the answer, perhaps followed by radiotherapy and chemotherapy. The cure rate, even in the advanced stage of the tumour, is about 80 per cent.

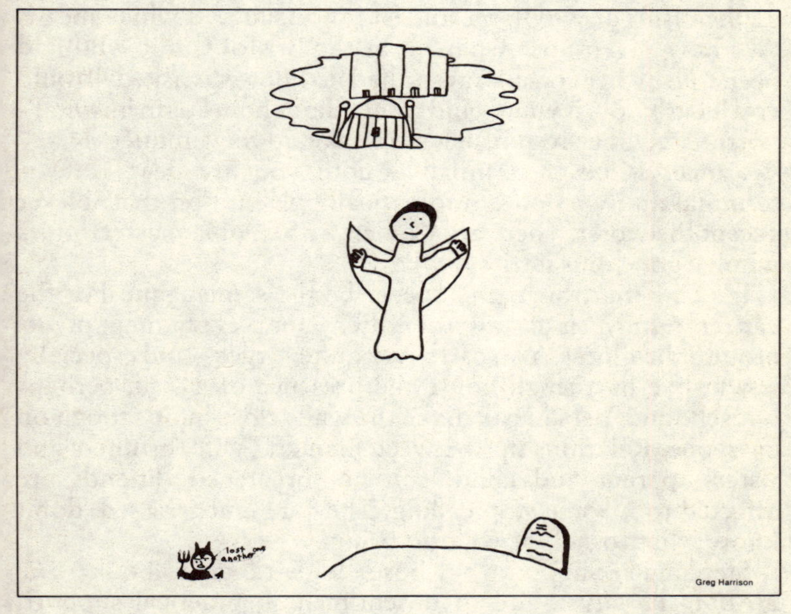

Greg Harrison

9
Home Again

Most cancer patients do not remain in hospital. They go home. Some to pick up the threads and get on with life. Some to be nursed by their families. Others are discharged with such euphemisms as 'Go home and sit in the sun' . . . which means 'We have given up'. A patient at the Bristol Clinic who had been told by her consultant she had no hope was asked 'Would you let us know if you would rather die at home or in hospital'! Fortunately, her response was to take up the gauntlet.

Cancer is never terminal – until you are dead. Life is terminal and we don't automatically give up on that. Never accept the worst. There are women with double mastectomies who've gone on safari.

It's true that things may never be the same again. For the cancer family finds, all too often, that everything pivots around the illness. You can never quite forget – and especially if you live in a small house the presence of a sick, perhaps housebound, person can make the walls close in. It's tough on everyone. Relationships between man and wife, brothers and sisters, parent and child, can be threatened. Friends are affected too. Some stop calling. They are embarrassed, don't know what to say, or what to bring.

Stephanie Simonton, whose wide-ranging book *The Healing Family* is full of unsentimental, practical support, talks of developing a Family Game plan. She talks of sustaining as near a normal pattern as possible . . . have friends in, go to your club, send the kids to discos. Take a regular walk, plenty of sleep, good food. Even well members of a family could find meditation and relaxation tapes a boon.

No one within a cancer family should become a martyr to the cause. Beware, too, she says, of taking over the patient's usual role within the family. Leave them in the driver's seat, making decisions and being involved in everyday life. There's a danger that sympathetic friends and family may become 'rescuers' and not helpers.

'Rescuers do not take care of their own needs, putting all their energy instead into caring for the patient. After weeks of self-neglect they can become angry.' One of the best ways for friends or relatives to avoid 'rescuing' is to focus more on their own needs. It is natural to want very much to help. But if that desire leads to rescuing, no matter how well intentioned, it may not be helpful. Instead it can defeat the patient's own efforts to work towards recovery. Family members who can, instead, support the patient and respect his autonomy will play an essential and very positive role.

Finding a balance is hard. The patient should never be allowed to dominate any group of family or of friends. This needs very sensitive handling because cancer or the drugs used in its care can sometimes cause dramatic changes in personality. These can rub off on everyone else. So if you feel tetchy, or sad, or scared, say so. Ask the patient to help. This is your world too.

Depression is common. Not so much the depression of the fear of death. This is honest-to-goodness depression at the way the illness is behaving. Feeling rotten, looking terrible, suffering pain are enough to make anyone fed up. Sometimes drugs lower defences and the heartache and failures of life — usually kept well in perspective — come flooding in. It's worth checking drugs and strengths with the doctor if this happens. Don't try too hard to jolly the patient along. Sympathise instead, agree that it's ghastly, and if possible find a distraction or ask the patient to say what would help. If the patient cries, hold his hand.

Touching is so important now. To the undemonstrative British, this is hard. Displays of physical affection are foreign. But a hand to hold, a cuddle or a gentle kiss can brighten any day. Closeness counts, cancer need not kill love.

Illness can also be a tool: it entitles us to be more demanding — to ask for love, or to say 'no'. It is not unusual for patients to 'go off' people, to refuse visitors and even to list those who are or are not wanted. There is in a sense a removal of taboos, no need now to worry about upsetting people with whom relationships were uneasy. These reactions often come from the deep subconscious. It is an exorcising of bad memories or a way of being angry with life. A sick person very often can't cope with being tactful or handling long-standing tricky relationships.

Equally, and more unkindly, a patient may refuse to see a close relative . . . a mother . . . or a son, just because they are too well-loved and the invalid can't bear to cause distress. If this happens, bring in a third party, or ask for help from the cancer counselling group who will advise. But don't be too soft. Even a cancer victim can stand a gentle ticking off. Of course, it is not always like this. Cancer can, fortunately, bring people closer, but it does help to understand when there's a variation in the pattern.

Much depends on how well or ill the patient is. Cancer sometimes generates a surprising amount of super-charged energy. Physical activity may not always be possible but if a patient wants to dig the garden, let them get on with it. Go out and join in. A day trip to Boulogne, a special holiday, some way-out clothes – all are helpful, not in the sense of a 'last fling' but because they make each day worth living and that is what it is all about. Things are certainly not all bad. Many cancer patients even claim they are glad – the experience caused them to revalue and enjoy life.

Cancer at Work

If the patient makes progress and is able to get out and about, the quicker a really normal life can be resumed the better.

It is very often difficult for a cancer patient to get – or even hold – a job. The reason is partly fear of unreliability but the stigma of the illness is still strong and very often people decide to hide the truth. Since there are many forms of cancer that do not show at all and some that simmer for years, to be penalised unnecessarily is hard. The person with cancer needs to feel needed and respected, not shunned. Managers tend to urge early retirement or prefer to pay sick pay if the colleague will stay at home. These are problems best tackled head on, maybe discussed at a staff meeting with the cancer patient present to assess exactly their capabilities, desires and potential contribution. Sometimes, people discover what was wrong with their working lives through cancer and with goodwill all round it can be put right for them and others.

Cancer Alone

Cancer can be itself an isolating, lonely illness. It may be that if you live by yourself you are better adapted to withstand loneliness, but no one should attempt to struggle on without asking for help. If Mahomet doesn't go to the mountain, then the mountain must go to Mahomet — no one can know you need them unless you say so.

This is the time for weaving a net around you — making use of local organisations, asking neighbours to shop, inviting friends in, even if they bring their own supper. Isolation only increases depression. Grow plants . . . buy a pet . . . have something to care for and to watch growing. There are people for whom solitude is right and that should be respected. But even they may need someone to get their Social Security or take the milk in.

Practicalities

Your social worker, health visitor or doctor should know all there is to know about the practical problems that face any family caring for a cancer patient whether bed-bound or mobile. All too often, this information has to be wrung from those in the know. The Red Cross will usually help with the loan of bed-pans, water beds, urinals and back rests. Your local Cancer Self Help Group will be able to put you in touch with someone who has been through the same mill and so knows where to go. The Lisa Sainsbury Foundation (see Useful Addresses) was established to assist families with material, day-to-day needs.

The problems confronting a cancer patient are sometimes much the same as those facing any long term invalid; they include weight loss, constipation or diarrhoea, dry mouth, insomnia, the general discomfort of being bed-bound and, above all, pain.

Weight Loss
The most balanced, nutritious diet in the world is useless if you can't eat it. It is counter productive to embark on a food regime that makes you and your family utterly miserable. On the

other hand, some cancer patients who become obsessive about diets do find that this gives them a framework, something to hang on to. So bear with such whims and, if necessary, learn to cook seaweed!

The combination of the cancer itself and the drugs controlling it may make any food taste disagreeable and if a patient is not attempting a change of diet, even favourite food can taste nasty. Often, too, there is difficulty in swallowing, dry mouth and an acute loss of appetite.

Points for the patient — and some for the cook:

- Eat when you feel hungry even if it is not a meal time
- Make the eating area pleasant and whenever possible get up for meals
- Keep snacks by your bed to nibble (raisins, dates)
- To increase appetite, try tart flavours . . . live yoghurt, a glass of white wine
- Marinate chicken, fish or meat in fruit juice or white wine
- Add plenty of herbs to meals
- Drink plenty of fluids but not with meals
- Chew slowly
- Rest before eating
- If you have sores under your dentures, do not wear dentures when you do not need them for eating
- If you have mouth or throat problems, be sure your doctor examines the area to see whether or not you need special medication
- If your mouth is dry, ask the doctor whether the medicines you are taking are causing the dryness
- Cold foods can sometimes be soothing. Add ice to fruit juice for extra coldness
- Use gravies and sauces on vegetables. Cook stews and casseroles, adding more liquids to make them softer
- Cut your meat up in small pieces. Use a blender (cook the food first and then put it in the blender to make it easy to eat)
- Choose soft foods such as mashed potatoes, yoghurt, scrambled or poached eggs, egg custards, ricotta cheese, puddings, jellies, creamy cereals, and macaroni cheese
- Stay away from foods that sting or burn such as citrus fruit juices and tomatoes. Fruits low in acid (bananas, canned

pears) and nectars (peach, pear, apricot) are easier to swallow. Use a little sugar to tone down acid or salty foods
- Rinse your mouth whenever you feel you need it — to remove debris, stimulate your gums, lubricate your mouth, or make it feel fresher. You can make a mouthwash from 1 teaspoon of salt to 1 quart of water (or 1 teaspoon of baking soda to 1 quart of water). A mixture of equal parts of glycerine and warm water is also effective. Do not use a commercial mouthwash without your doctor's permission. Artificial saliva sprays are obtainable from most chemists
- Stay away from strong fumes such as cleaning solutions and paints.

Constipation

This is commonly due to drugs and general inactivity and although an increased fibre intake can help it is not always appropriate in, for instance, cases of colon cancer. Enemas, which help to remove toxicity, can be beneficial and there are a number of gentle herbal laxatives on the market.

Diarrhoea

In addition to drugs, there are foods which help to control diarrhoea — bananas, rice, cooked fruit and vegetables minus skins, or seeds. Diarrhoea causes a loss of vital potassium so include potassium-rich items in any diet.

Insomnia

Sleeplessness can become a nightmare and somehow the harder a patient tries to overcome it the worse the problem. Especially if there is a need to doze during the day, the long, lonely nights can become a source of terrible distress. Sleeping tablets may well be necessary; an alcoholic nightcap (not at the same time) is an alternative, as is favourite music tapes on a personal stereo system. But all in all, one of the hardest lessons to learn about insomnia is not to fight it too hard . . . read, do jigsaws, write a diary. Regular meditation is also helpful.

General Comfort — the Steps to Take

Frequent changes of position are important if the patient is confined to bed. This can be a real problem for the family if daily heavy lifting is involved. It is vital that everyone should take great care of their own health. Aromatic oil massage and relaxation and rest are as essential for the carers as the patient, or there is a real danger of strain and tiredness causing back trouble.

Sheepskin pads are a boon to prevent bedsores, and a cardboard box with a hole cut out for the legs makes an efficient means of raising bedclothes off tender limbs. An adjustable hospital bed can sometimes be hired and this makes changing of sheets and altering foot levels much easier. Don't forget a bell by the bed and, if possible, a rope tied to the footrest so that the invalid can pull himself up.

A humidifier or steam kettle can sometimes help the dry atmosphere in centrally-heated rooms. Air ionisers are also useful. These restore the balance of positive and negative ions in the atmosphere and are available in a number of shapes and sizes from health centres and other specialist sources.

Incontinence

This is feared by most of us as the ultimate degradation and it is wise for the family to remember that, however hard caring for incontinence may seem, it is far worse for the patient. The shock can cause much distress and tearfulness. There are many aids to make life easier for you all, including not only special bed pads but disposable underwear for men and women which helps boost confidence especially at night and saves over-frequent changing of bed clothes. But when changes are imperative, get organised beforehand and keep them speedy.

Bed Baths

Usually these are the responsibility of the health visitor, but it is useful to be able to manage on your own.

Prepare washbasin, warm water, flannels, towels, soap and toilet articles beforehand. An extra cotton blanket or large bathtowel will be needed to cover the patient when you remove the gown or pyjamas. Expose only the part of the body to be washed. Place a towel under each part as you wash it, dry thoroughly and cover. Remember to support the patient's arms and legs directly under the joints during the bath.

Allow the patient to do as much for himself or herself as is safely possible.

Always follow the same order starting with the eyes, face, neck, ears, chest and abdomen, far arm, near arm, hands, far leg, near leg, feet, back, buttocks, genitals. You'll notice this order is designed to use the cleanest water on the most sensitive areas. Another method used recommends: face, arms and trunk to hips, back and buttocks, legs, feet, and genitals. Bath water can be changed before the back, buttocks and genitals are washed. Hands and feet can be washed in the basin. Allow the patient to wash the genitals if he or she is able to do so.

Coping with Pain

Britain leads the world in pain control of all kinds. The United States is five years behind. But even that spot of news doesn't help if you wake in the night, gripped by the panic of pain tearing you to shreds and don't know where to turn for help. No mind over matter then. No visualising fakirs on beds of nails. Happiness is the pill bottle.

Generally speaking, cancer creeps up quietly from behind. It does not hurt. But that is not always the case and when it is bad it can be very, very bad. In Chris Williams' book *All about cancer*, Susan Williams writes:

> One of the most important reasons for failure to control pain is the lack of appreciation by doctors that it is not a simple physical sensation. As well as the physical perception of pain, there is the emotional reaction to it. Perception of pain and pain thresholds are closely linked to mood and morale and a good relationship between patient and doctor is very helpful. Pain is extremely difficult to evaluate. It varies from person to person . . . some can tolerate a lot more than others.

The answer, ideally, is to prevent pain from getting a hold. If you expect pain – pain you will feel. So, forget the fear that causes the tension that brings on the pain. The first step is to encourage the patient to remain absorbed in activities or engrossing pursuits at all times . . . fishing, walking, writing, watching TV. Pain seems to be evaporated by such distraction.

Second – lend a willing ear. Physical pain can be caused by suppressing feelings. It is the mind screaming. Consequently, a priest, healer or confidante discreetly taking on the role of 'confessor' can be therapeutic.

Third – pain is often caused by the treatment, not the cancer, and this is hard to handle. It is best to discuss and understand progress with the doctors and perhaps suggest the use of visualisation techniques to side-step the pain.

But if all this hasn't worked, the mind is tired and bodily resistance low, what then? In theory, no one should have to suffer. It is your right to have pain controlled. But in reality it is otherwise. Pain control, which began about 15 years ago in Seattle, USA, should exist in all 14 Regional Health Authorities, but it doesn't. Instead, there are varying degrees of help available, from the single-handed anaesthetist in the general hospital to the superbly caring expertise of the specialist nurses at home and in hospices. GPs are sadly ignorant about the latest NHS pain relief services or holistic techniques.

There are two types of pain – acute and chronic. Acute pain should be treatable by the GP, whereas chronic pain, which is persistent, mounting and long lasting, may need specialist help. So, what to do? The orthodox say there are three basic ways of controlling pain, and all should be supervised.

1 Drugs: beginning with the best known, aspirin or para-cetamol (avoid aspirin if you are on chemotherapy as it damages the platelets) through to Distalgesic, Napsalgesic, Codis, Paracodal and DF118 or Paramol 118 for more persistent pain and, finally, the narcotics, opium-based, for severe pain; the latter cannot be dispensed by a chemist as they are addictive and, in the long run, lower tolerance to pain. They can be given orally, but also by injection in urgent cases.
2 Nerve blocks: given by an anaesthetist in hospital to damage the nerve and block off the pain.
3 Central modulation: this is the use of hypnosis and Biofeedback to make the brain cancel pain. Peripheral modulation is when the body nerves are stimulated by massage or acupuncture (this is sometimes used in even an orthodox hospital) along with transcutaneous stimulation by electrical impulses across the skin.

Such help should be available in any hospital, but increasingly it is possible to administer pain relief at home – either through the Pain Clinic or the Hospice organisations. Marie Curie Foundation and Macmillan nurses are trained in pain control; in all cases ask your GP — or the hospital oncologist.

So often, patients long for relief from pain but not for loss of consciousness. They want to remain alert and, with skill, this is perfectly possible today. They may become tired . . . but not unconscious. Always say exactly what is needed.

Sometimes doctors ask patients to keep a log as this is very helpful towards the understanding of pain especially as it is so hard to define. It also keeps the patient involved in his progress. Overleaf is a pilot questionnaire used by the SW Thames Regional Cancer Organisation, which is part of the Royal Marsden Hospital.

Most of the complementary therapies offer help with pain control, without drugs. Acupuncture, in particular, is widely used — in fact, it became known first to the British public as an anaesthetic enabling patients to watch their own operations. All forms of relaxation and meditation, too, offer release if the patient is able to participate but not everyone finds this easy. Osteopathic release techniques and massage are also helpful, especially after an operation.

The Final Stage of Growth — The Hospice Movement

The words hospice and hospital share the same origins. In Rome nearly 1600 years ago when the Latin *hospes* meant both guest and host, Fabiola, a disciple of St Jerome, founded a refuge for pilgrims returning from Africa. Then and in medieval times the role of these places was as a fusion of medical and spiritual shelter. Hospital and hospitality meant one and the same; all were given shelter, the poor, the sick, the homeless.

It is not a coincidence that the hospice ideal has been revived in the last 20 years. A new seeking for spiritual values and an increasing openness and understanding about death, has led to a far greater sensitivity towards the needs of the dying. Modern hospices are places of transit, where terminal patients are not manipulated by artificial means but are gently helped

NAME ___________________________

ADDRESS _________________________

If you are in pain we can treat it properly with the right medicine given it is at the right time for you. To help us know what is the best medicine for you to have, I would like you to fill in this simple diary whenever you get pain. I really want to know when you get pain, *where* you get it and *how bad it is.*

First of all, tell me where your pain is by marking it on the two diagrams below.

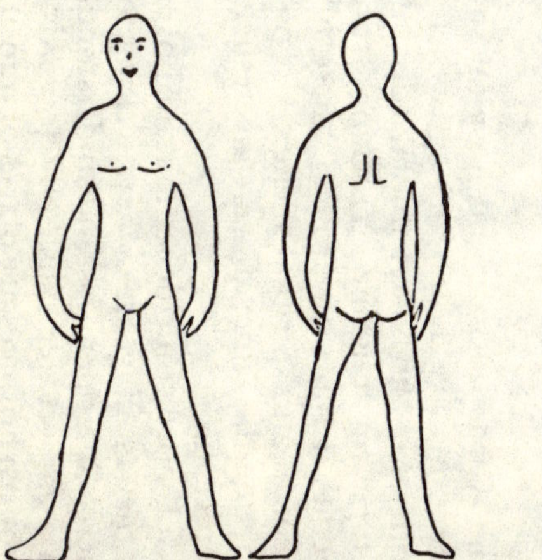

LEVEL OF PAIN

Example only:-

0	1	2	3	4	5
NO PAIN	MILD PAIN	MODERATE PAIN	SEVERE PAIN	VERY SEVERE PAIN	INTOLERABLE OVERWHELMING PAIN

This diagram shows different levels of pain. Each time you are aware of pain, mark on the line on the diary below* how bad your pain is. If you grade it 2 or more, please contact me or your family doctor so that we can then discuss a better way of treating it.

THE DIARY – you can fill this in when you get pain. Please be careful to make a note of the *TIME* and the *DATE* when you do.

DATE	TIME	WHERE IS THE WORST PAIN?	HOW BAD IS THE WORST PAIN?	WHAT TIME DID YOU TAKE YOUR LAST PAINKILLER?	WHAT WAS THE DOSE?	ARE THERE ANY OTHER COMMENTS YOU WISH TO MAKE?
			*0 1 2 3 4 5			
			*0 1 2 3 4 5			
			*0 1 2 3 4 5			
			*0 1 2 3 4 5			
			*0 1 2 3 4 5			

DATE	TIME	WHERE IS THE WORST PAIN?	HOW BAD IS THE WORST PAIN?	WHAT TIME DID YOU TAKE YOUR LAST PAINKILLER?	WHAT WAS THE DOSE?	ARE THERE ANY OTHER COMMENTS YOU WISH TO MAKE?
			*0 1 2 3 4 5			
			*0 1 2 3 4 5			
			*0 1 2 3 4 5			
			*0 1 2 3 4 5			
			*0 1 2 3 4 5			
			*0 1 2 3 4 5			
			*0 1 2 3 4 5			
			*0 1 2 3 4 5			

PERSONAL DIARY
DATE OF ISSUE
/   /

CONSULTANT:

TEL. NO:-

FAMILY DOCTOR:

TEL. NO:-

PLEASE TAKE THIS CARD WITH YOU WHENEVER
YOU GO TO THE OUT-PATIENTS CLINIC OR TO
YOUR FAMILY DOCTOR.

through that 'final stage of growth' as Elizabeth Kubler Ross has called it. They are sunny, well-equipped and radiating warmth, staffed by specially trained nurses. Increasingly they can also be places of rest and restoration and many patients return home, often much better.

The pioneer of this work in Britain was Dame Cicely Saunders, the founder of St Christopher's Hospice in London. The success of her tireless efforts was built on a love story. When she was just 29 in 1947 she fell in love with a young Jewish cancer patient, David Tasma. On his death, he bequeathed £500 to help her found the first purpose-built hospital for the dying, in London. 'I'll be a window in your home,' he told her.

St Christopher's was opened at last in 1967 and became a model for the world. Today it operates not only 'the village' where patients live and are cared for in a superbly equipped but informal atmosphere – families and pets are welcome at all times – there is also a Home Care service. The families of those who wish to die at home are very often overcome with fear. The missionary role of St Christopher's as a teaching hospital is much in demand and it provides an invaluable source of literature and information for the public, not only about Dame Cicely's approach but about coping with death and bereavement and the work of other hospices.

There are now over 100 hospices in Britain – some purpose-built – others, like St Joseph's in London adapted from Victorian premises. Far from being places of despair, they are richly rewarding to those who go there. The sharing of the experience of dying is often a tremendous comfort. Dame Cicely has said 'This is a place of meeting. Physical and spiritual, doing and accepting, giving and receiving, all have to be brought together. The dying need the community, its help and fellowship, the community needs the dying to make it think of eternal issues.' No talk here, or in any hospice, of euthanasia: 'For anyone to contemplate mercy killing would be a poor reflection on their nurses or doctors.'

Understandably, there is a religious base for any hospice, but patients belong to all faiths – and none. 'The courtesy of the Orient and the traditional hospitality of Abraham are as much a part of the hospice vision as Christian liturgy,' wrote Sandol Stoddard in *The Hospice Movement*.

The decision about whether to die at home or in a hospice may be the choice of the patient but may well have to be taken by an anxious family, desperate to do the best for a loved one in frightening and unfamiliar circumstances. The amount of help available for terminal care at home varies greatly in different parts of Britain, but it is improving. No one should be afraid to seek the support of a domiciliary 'hospice at home' team because there is comfort for all in the daily arrival of a nurse who can ease the burden a little. She can become a friend to the patient. Equally, she is a source of tremendous strength for relatives and friends who are worn out, often to breaking point, by lifting, bed changing, feeding and simply watching a loved one so ill. Tempers are frayed and tension high.

Hospice care has developed in a number of different ways:

• *Patient Hospice Units*, such as St Joseph's. These are financed mainly by charitable income and some offer a home care service. There are also independent units administered by a charity, such as Sue Ryder Homes and the Marie Curie Memorial Foundation, which has 4,000 trained and auxiliary nurses available night and day nationwide for home care.

• *Macmillan Continuing Care Homes*, built in the grounds of National Health hospitals from capital provided initially by the National Society for Cancer Relief and taken over now by the NHS.

• *Macmillan Mini Units*, two-bedded wards with a visitor's room attached to community hospitals in Wales. Again, built and equipped by the National Society for Cancer Relief and run by the NHS.

• *Continuing Care Wards*, in NHS hospitals.

• *Support Teams* and symptom control teams within NHS hospitals. These are peripatetic teams offering a supportive and advisory service within the hospital.

Help from: St Christopher's Hospice; St Joseph's Hospice (for both, see Useful Addresses). There are also centres for peace and quiet where cancer patients and/or their families can recover their strength for a short stay: Claridge House; Burrswood; Harmony House (for all three, see Useful Addresses).

A Time to Die

After every party the guests must depart.

Kothari

Acceptance of death does not necessarily mean it is around the corner. Hope springs eternal. But if there comes a time – either because a cancer has recurred or, perhaps, because the patient is becoming too ill to get up or care for himself, there are some who accept that this is 'a time to die'. A time for tying ends, tackling unfinished business. It is then the role of those around to help that process gently . . . a hard task when the patient is a loved and elderly relative, agonising when the patient is young and the parting shatters a family. But the truth is that under such pressures, unsuspected qualities can be drawn to the surface.

Talking about dying is not morbid. Nor does it indicate that the patient has given up. Normally, says Stephanie Simonton, 'as a patient explores questions about pain and fear and incapacity, his anxiety significantly decreases . . . this confidence frequently gives him the renewed energy to move back toward the living . . . he has seen that he can handle the worst that can happen; now he is free to move between two possibilities.' But it is very important that when the patient wants to discuss his own mortality, the family goes along with him, one pace behind. They must try, however hard, to let him lead the way and so retain his dignity.

In some ways, like Christmas or having visitors to stay, the thought of mortality engenders the need to have a good clear up. Sorting papers, organising family finances, even discussing wills, can be curiously therapeutic. There are some who like to take photographs, a memory for the album, others who keep a diary. Decisions such as funerals and place of burial, once made, can be a huge weight from a family's mind. If such things sound macabre or even flippant in cold blood, they are immensely comforting at the time.

Sadly there can be a problem for cancer patients about donating a body for research. The shock – and even a sense of shame – that it may not be acceptable is hard to face but the possibility is there and it is wise to be prepared.

The dying process too, though it is more often than not a gentle slipping away, does not always follow the text books.

Families are run down and tired to the point of collapse; there can be arguments and bedside tensions, uncharacteristic quarrelling over petty things. This, in itself, should not cause you distress for it is natural and will pass.

For most people, confronted with death in the family, belief and faith are inescapable. For believers of every faith there is support and counsel from their religious leaders. For those without a faith, this is not so and, however composed, however at peace with their understanding of life and death, there can be unexpected practical dilemmas for the family left behind. Probably there's a need for a final farewell, a tying of ends, yet a Christian service does not feel appropriate. Families in this situation will find that the Humanist Association and the Quakers can be kind and understanding. Both can help with arrangements that are spiritual in atmosphere but not aligned to a particular creed.

Beautiful music, poetry and readings by friends can make a moving and very personal tribute which can even be arranged in the family home, before, after or during the cremation.

Most Eastern philosophies see dying as a vehicle for awakening. Ram Dass is a past Professor of Psychology at Harvard University, a man who has written a great deal about giving life to the death process.

> At the moment of death each moment is the total thing you have. This moment is it, now this moment, now this moment and in moments you will drop your body and it will be just another moment. But how conscious we are of that moment, which is the result of the moment before it and the moment before it will decide what happens subsequently in the next moment which has to do with what is called reincarnation. So what will happen to you next will be a function of how you go through that doorway.

Aldous Huxley wrote in *Island* a poignant description of a man helping his wife to die.

> Lightly, my darling, lightly. Even when it comes to dying. Nothing ponderous, or portentous or emphatic. No rhetoric, no tremolos, no self conscious persona putting on its celebrated imitation of Christ, or Goethe, or Little Nell. And of course, no theology, no metaphysics. Just the fact of dying and the fact of clear light. So throw away all your baggage and go forward. There are quick-sands all about you sucking at your feet, trying to suck you down into fear, self pity and despair. That's why you must walk so lightly . . . so now you can let go my darling.

10
Life After Cancer

Families who live through cancer – whether or not death finally came – are changed, often transformed, by the experience. They know now that tomorrow is not forever. Almost without exception, cancer victims who survive feel enriched. If a child who was within days of death and suffered appallingly from drastic medical treatments and then recovered can say 'It really made me grow up', the same is true for many adults.

Of course, responses to bereavement vary enormously and are often unintelligible or even shocking to the outsider. Parents who have lost a child may be hurt that the siblings appear unconcerned. Those grieving most may put on the brightest face but grieve long, whereas the family that mourns loudest may be on its feet speedily. Not for nothing do West Indians wail . . . or did Lancashire folk hold a wake. These are devices for letting go. Essential now is tolerance and freedom – the bereaved must be allowed to react as they feel the need. They must feel free and only very gently guided from outside.

For many, clinging to the familiar routine is a vital security when the world has fallen apart. Women, in particular, can be very vulnerable when a loved one has died, especially if there has been a long and tiring time of nursing. They fall in love easily and there should be no guilt about this, only caution, for the reasons are seldom sound.

Try not to struggle alone – for, curiously enough, this is a time when friends can appear to fall away. With the best will in the world, their intention is to leave the mourner in peace, but the result is a sense of abandonment. The agony of eating alone, Saturday shopping or Sunday walks in the park are beyond their understanding, and whereas a couple are company for a meal or a night at the pub a single man or woman is often odd one out. These are the problems shared by all bereaved but there are ways forward and there is much experienced help and wise counsel to draw on, not least from your own cancer care group. Most important now is not to neglect the quality of your life.

Try to remember these wise words:

Life does not cease to be funny when people die, any more than it ceases to be serious when people laugh.

George Bernard Shaw

Laughter is a kind of spiritual jogging. An evening with Woody Allen or half an hour of Basil Fawlty really is a 'tonic'. For, just as emotional tensions have negative effects on body chemistry and depress the proper functioning of the adrenal glands and the endocrine system, so a hearty laugh can have the reverse effect. Humour is at all times a powerful therapy.

Of course, there must be many families for whom talk of humour, in the context of cancer, may seem callous, unthinkable. But if cancer itself is to be seen as an integral part of being alive, then laughter and its positive powers must have as important a role at all times. This is not a new idea: 400 years ago, Richard Burton wrote in *The Anatomy of Melancholy* 'Humour purges the blood making the body young, lively and fit for any manner of employment.' Kant and Freud both revered laughter as a therapy.

Norman Cousins, former writer and senior lecturer in medicine at the University of California, discovered just how important and wrote a bestseller on his discoveries – *The Anatomy of an Illness*. It is about his own 'terminal' illness and his belief that the human mind can mobilise the body's own ability to combat disease – and if not always to conquer it, at the very least to improve the quality of life remaining.

Working as a team with his doctor, he devised a programme which included massive doses of vitamin C and equal doses of laughter. 'Nothing is less funny than being flat on your back with all the bones in your spine and joints hurting', he admitted. But a series of *Candid Camera* television films and some Marx Bros movies produced belly laughter which, he declared, had an anaesthetic effect which brought him at least two pain-free hours and a hospital room to himself, well away from other patients.

Carefully logging his progress, Norman Cousins went

through a week. At the end of the eighth day, he was moving his thumbs without pain and the granular nodules on his neck and the backs of his hands were beginning to shrink. Some months later he returned to work, was riding and playing the piano and his mobility has improved yearly.

Norman Cousins chose a dramatic path to recovery. But good humour can be woven into the fabric of everyday living, so that it becomes simply doing what comes naturally. Norman Cousins writes of Dr Schweitzer, 'Albert Schweitzer employed humour as a form of equatorial therapy, a way of reducing the temperatures and the humidity and the tensions . . . it was so artistic that one had the feeling he regarded it almost as a musical instrument.' Laughter at dinner was probably the most important course and staff were rejuvenated by the wryness of his humour. Humour at Lambaréné was vital nourishment.

Was Norman Cousins the beneficiary of a mammoth adventure in self-administered placebos? Maybe – but no matter. There is nothing wrong in the placebo effect if it works.

Even death, however devastating, can be eventually a creative experience for those left behind. Many people find they are drawn to crusade energetically for a cancer cause, to raise money for a scanner or work for the local self help group. Others decide to start a hospice – or write a book. For death can always be seen as an end – or a beginning.

Family doctor Ian Pearce, who is much respected in the medical world, understands first-hand what it is like to cope with cancer. He says: 'If there is a message shining through the cancer story it must surely be the age old and oft repeated law: "Thou shalt not live by bread alone".' It is simply not enough merely to organise the material side of life. Emotional comfort and spiritual satisfaction are equally necessary. We need a sense of direction and purpose in life; an intuitive understanding that, even if we cannot perceive it, we are going somewhere. All true healing, whether of cancer or of any other disease, can only come when these conditions obtain. Therefore our approach must be truly holistic – that is to say it must operate on all levels.

It could be tempting in the first flush of discovery to select one of the great range of therapies and go along with that, and to discard the remainder. Such a course is almost invariably disastrous! All therapies, including those of orthodox medicine, are valid at their own level – and only at their own level. But each one of us exists upon a variety of different levels, all of which are affected in cancer, either as a contributory factor causing the disease or as a secondary consequence of it, and help is needed at each of these levels. The cardinal feature of the new approach is that it recognises these different levels and endeavours to help the patient wherever help is needed. It also understands that the patient must be encouraged to play an active role in the healing process, rather than adopt an attitude of passive submission.

Crucial to the healing of cancer is the understanding that it is saying something to the sufferer. It is telling the patient that something about his or her life is wrong and needs to be changed. But if the sufferer will accept this need, if, instead of asking 'Why should this have to happen to me?' he or she will ask 'What is this telling me about my life?', then a start can be made upon setting things right. The essence of healing is transformation, and the task of the healer is to assist in that transformation and to maintain life while it comes into being. All therapies, whether orthodox or complementary, are subsidiary to this basic requirement, and all must work within the natural framework of the self-healing powers of the body.

The plea, therefore, is for an end to aggression and confrontation: for the positive sharing of knowledge and skill between all members of the healing professions, be they surgeon or healer without pride or prejudice: for the recognition that the healing act is a partnership between the patient and the therapist(s), and that unless each play their part honestly and to the maximum of their ability, nothing is possible.

Cancer is no more cruel, no more devastating than many other illnesses, but since it is so greatly feared let it become a shop window for a positive approach to health – in which the important factor is how and why we live, not why we die. This is the way to undermine cancer's hold upon us.

> Life may be understood looking backwards
> But life must be lived looking forwards.
>
> *Anon.*

Glossary

Compiled by Sally Evemy

Ablative Therapy A treatment to totally remove or eradicate part of the body.

Acupuncture An ancient therapy evolved in China, involving the insertion of fine needles into points along channels or 'meridians' of energy in the body, in order to manipulate body energies for healing.

Acute Coming sharply to a crisis – opposite of Chronic.

Adenocarcinoma A cancer starting in glandular tissue.

Adjuvant Therapy A secondary treatment which usually follows surgery and involves chemotherapy or radiotherapy.

Adrenalectomy Removal of an adrenal gland.

Aetiology The study of the cause of a disease.

Aflatoxin One of a number of toxic carcinogenic substances which may contaminate badly stored products, notably peanuts.

Allopathic The system of medicine using drugs of a non-homoeopathic nature: that is, all 'orthodox' forms of drug therapy based on a mechanistic model of the human body.

Alopecia Loss of hair which can be caused by some types of chemotherapy and radiation to the scalp. It is nearly always temporary.

Alteratives Name, in herbalism, given to those herbs used when dealing with tumours which cleanse and normalise. See also Anti-Neoplastics.

Alternative All those branches of medicine not currently espoused by 'orthodox' or mechanistic medical science.

Amenorrhoea Loss of normal menstruation or periods.

Amino Acid The building material from which protein is made by the body.

Amygdalin Soluble glycoside extracted from bitter almonds or apricot kernels and found in many other seeds and berries, water-cress, bean sprouts and lentils: sometimes known as vitamin B17.

Anaemia Lack of red cells in the blood which causes tiredness, shortness of breath and pallor.

Anaesthesia Total or partial loss of sensation (especially pain) and/or consciousness. An anaesthetic is a substance that produces anaesthesia.

Analgesic Medicine given (by mouth, injection or suppository) to control pain.

Androgen A male hormone.

Anorexia Absence of appetite or desire.

Anthroposophy A philosophical school owing much to the holistic teachings of Rudolph Steiner (1861–1925) on a number of subjects, with a developed medical science based on a subtle understanding of the medicinal uses of plants and minerals.

Antibiotic A drug – for example, penicillin – that is used to treat diseases caused by bacteria. Antibiotics are not effective against diseases caused by viruses.

Antibody A protein produced by the body's immune system in response to an intruder. Antibodies serve to render intruders harmless.

Antigen A protein that serves to identify intruders that have invaded the body. Antigens provoke the immune system to form antibodies.

Anti-neoplastics Name, in herbalism, given to those herbs used when dealing with tumours which block new growth. See also Alteratives.

Arteriogram A special test to outline an artery, involving insertion of a fine catheter and use of contrast dye and X-rays.

Aspirate To suck off fluid with a syringe.

Astrocytoma The commonest cancer that develops in the brain in adults.

Axilla The armpit.

Bacteria Single-celled organisms formed in the shape of rods, spheres and spirals. Some bacteria are helpful to the body. Others cause disease – for example, tuberculosis.

Barium A natural metal, the sulphate of which is used as a contrast medium for X-rays.

Benign A term used to describe tissue or a tumour which is not malignant or cancerous and which, therefore, does not spread.

Bilateral Pertaining to both sides.

Biochemical Relating to chemical or physico-chemical processes and products involved in life phenomena of plants and animals.

Biodynamic A variant of organic farming, based on indications given by Rudolf Steiner, in which supposed terrestrial and cosmic influences are taken into account.

Bioenergetic Conversion of energy in biologic functions, as in food-sugar-energy.

Biofeedback Technique of using feedback of a normally automatic bodily response to a stimulus, in order to acquire voluntary control of the response.

Biopsy The surgical removal of a piece of tissue for examination under a microscope.

Blood Count A count of the number of white blood cells, red blood cells and platelets in a sample of blood.

B-Lymphocytes White blood cells from bone marrow.

Body Scan Another name for a CAT scan – a special X-ray that gives very detailed pictures.

Bone Marrow Spongy tissue in the middle of bones that makes blood cells.

Bone Marrow Biopsy and Aspiration The removal of a small amount of bone marrow for examination under a microscope. This is done by pushing a fine needle (after local anaesthetic) into the pelvis or the breast bone.

Bowel The lower digestive tract, comprising the small (duodenum, jejeunum and ileum) and large (colon and rectum) intestines.

Brain Scan A way of examining the brain after injecting a small amount of a radioactive 'dye'.

Bronchoscopy Examination of the air passages with a flexible instrument called a bronchoscope.

BSE Breast self-examination.

Cachexia A general weakening of the body.

Calorie A measurement of energy – often as contained in food.

Cancer A general term for more than a hundred diseases where there is uncontrolled growth of cells which spread and, if untreated, eventually lead to death.

Carbohydrate A group of substances in food, including sugars, dextrins, starches and celluloses.

Carcinogen A substance that can cause or help cause cancer.

Carcinoma A cancer that develops from cells called epithelial cells. These cells are present in the skin, lungs, glands, gastro-intestinal tract, and urinary tract. Cancers that develop in these places are called carcinomas and are the commonest type of cancer.

Carotene The plant form of vitamin A.

Cartesian Philosophy named after René Descartes based on the sharp division of body and soul.

Catalyst A substance which by its presence speeds up or slows down a chemical reaction but which remains unchanged by the process.

Catheter A slender tube that can be passed into a blood vessel, or through a canal. Catheters are used to introduce fluids into the body (for example, blood) or withdraw fluids (for example, urine).

CAT Scan A computerised X-ray system that gives very detailed pictures.

Cell The smallest unit of life. All living tissue is composed of cells.

Cervical Smear Scraping of cells from the neck of the womb (cervix) for examination under a microscope.

Cervix Neck of the uterus or womb.

Ch'i or Qi In Chinese medicine, name given to body energies.

Chemotherapy The use of drugs to treat cancer.

Cholecystogram A special test relating to the gall bladder and involving contrast dye and X-ray.

Cholesterol A normal constituent of all animal fats and oils.

Chronic Lingering, or lasting – opposite of Acute.

Cirrhosis Chronic, progressive disease of the liver.

Clinical Investigations Investigations in which doctors test a new drug or treatment on human patients. Also called clinical tests and field tests.

Cobalt A radioactive substance used in radiotherapy. Cobalt produces gamma rays, a form of radiation very much like X-rays.

Co-carcinogen A chemical that is not in itself cancer-causing, but that can somehow provoke another chemical to cause cancer.

Colon The large bowel.

Colonoscopy The use of a flexible instrument to examine the entire large bowel.

Colostomy An operation to bring the bowel (colon) up to the abdominal wall so that faeces may be collected in a special bag.

Colposcopy Examination of the neck of the womb with a magnifying instrument passed into the vagina.

Combination Chemotherapy The use of several drugs given together to treat cancer.

Combined Modality Treatment The use of more than one type of anti-cancer treatment (surgery, radiotherapy and chemotherapy) together.

Complementary All the 'alternative' forms of medicine – acupuncture, osteopathy, homoeopathy, etc. – as practised with the emphasis on cooperation with and support for the orthodox forms of medicine.

Consultant Senior hospital doctor.

Contagious A contagious disease is one that can be passed from one person to another.

Contrast Film Medium used to show differences in X-ray absorption.

Craniopharyngioma A tumour of the pituitary gland at the base of the brain.

CT Scan See CAT scan.

Cure The elimination of disease, so that a patient recovers his health.

Since cancer may appear to be cured when it is not, doctors talk about cancer cures in terms of years: 'a five year cure', 'a six year cure', etc.

Cyst A small, benign sac that contains fluid or semi-solid material.

Cystoscopy Use of an instrument passed through the passage from the bladder to examine the inside of the bladder.

Cytogenic Encouraging new cell growth.

Cytology The study of cells.

Cytoplasm The 'soupy' material that surrounds the nucleus of a cell.

Dehydration Loss of fluid.

Detoxification A process whereby substances foreign to the body are changed to compounds more easily eliminated. Popularly thought of as 'cleansing' of the body.

DNA (Deoxyribonucleic Acid) The genetic material in the centre of a cell which controls its growth, division and function.

Diagnosis A medical identification of a disease in a patient.

Dialysis The use of a kidney machine to remove impurities from a patient's blood.

Differentiated Cells Mature cells that perform a specific function in the body – for example, blood cells, skin cells or bone cells.

Diuretic Substance causing increased excretion of urine.

Dysuria Pain on passing urine.

Ecologist One who studies the effect of surroundings or environment on an organism.

Electrons Particles of negative electricity found within atoms.

Electromagnetic Magnetic field produced by an electric current.

Embryo The product of conception, up to the third month of pregnancy.

Encapsulated Term for tumour in a shell-like capsule.

Endocrine Gland Gland that secretes hormones into the bloodstream.

Endocrine Therapy The use of hormones to treat a disease.

Endometrium Lining of the womb that is shed with each period.

Endorphine A substance with morphine-like properties secreted by the brain.

Endoscopy The use of a hollow instrument to examine the inside of different parts of the body.

Enema A rectal infusion for therapeutic or nutritive purposes.

Environment Circumstances of life of person or society.

Enzyme A catalytic substance formed by living cells and having a specific action in promoting chemical changes.

Epidemiology The study of the geographical distribution of disease.

Epidural Passing a syringe needle through the fibrous outer covering of the spinal cord, for purposes of injection.

ESR (Erythrocyte sedimentation rate) Warning sign in blood test when red cells sink to the bottom.

Euthanasia Mercy killing.

Excisional Biopsy Total surgical removal of tissue to be examined.

Fermentation The breakdown of complex substances under the influence of enzymes or ferments.

Fibre Woody material in food that remains undigested, essential in its bulky scouring action to the health of the bowels.

Fibrocystic Disease A benign breast condition in which there is overgrowth of fibrous tissue often combined with formation of cysts.

Fibroids Lumps of fibrous endometrial tissue found in the womb.

Fibroma Benign tumour found in fibrous connective tissue.

Fistulae Opening of a wound or abscess, usually transmitting pus or fluid.

Fluoride A salt which appears naturally but is also a by-product of industrial processes.

Frozen Section A rapid way of examining a biopsy to see if it contains cancer; a result is available straight away so that a suitable operation can be planned.

Gamma Rays High energy radiation.

Ganglion A benign tumour-like growth usually formed on tendon sheath or joint capsule.

Gastroscopy The use of a flexible instrument, which is swallowed, to examine the inside of the stomach and upper part of the small bowel.

Genetic Concerning biological inheritance.

Geopathic Stress Electromagnetic and energic stresses deriving from local geology and terrestrial radiations, now extended to include man-made electromagnetic stresses from electricity, microwaves, radio waves and radioactivity.

Glioblastoma A highly malignant brain cancer in adults.

Glycolysis The breakdown of carbohydrate in tissue to pyruvic or lactic acid; the means whereby cancer cells obtain energy when they no longer use oxygen.

Granulocytes (Neutrophils) Infection-fighting cells in the blood.

Gynaecologist A doctor who specialises in the treatment of diseases of the female reproductive tract.

Haematologist A doctor who specialises in diseases of the blood and bone marrow.

Haemorrhage Heavy, uncontrolled bleeding.

Haematuria Blood in the urine.

Hepatoma A primary cancer of the liver.

Herbalist Medical practitioner using the medicinal properties of plants and foods for therapeutic effect.

Heredity The transmission from parent to child of characteristics that are determined by the genes.

Histology The study of tissues to diagnose disease.

Holism The belief that mind, body and spirit cannot be regarded as separate entities.

Homoeopathy A system of medicine using minute doses of substances which would produce, in a healthy person, the same symptoms as the disease for which they are administered.

Hormone A chemical substance that circulates in the blood and causes changes in the body.

Hormone Receptor Assay A special test to see if a tumour contains special receptor sites that indicate that it is likely to respond to hormone therapy.

Hormone Therapy The use of hormones to treat a disease.

Hospice A hospital specially equipped for the care of dying patients.

Houseman Junior hospital doctor.

Hyperalimentation The infusion or drip of highly nutritious fluids containing protein and lots of calories into a vein.

Hypernephroma A cancer of the kidney in adults.

Hyperthermic Therapeutic high temperature. Often induced by hot baths.

Hypophysectomy Surgical removal of the pituitary gland.

Hysterectomy An operation to remove the womb (uterus).

Iatrogenic Damage produced by the physician or by drugs.

Ileum Lower part of the small bowel.

Ileostomy An operation to bring the small bowel (ileum) up to the abdominal wall so that faeces can be collected in a bag.

Immune System The body's defence mechanisms against disease.

Immunity Protection against a specific disease. The body normally creates immunity by forming antibodies against bacteria and viruses that cause disease.

Immuno-Suppressive Treatment by drug or radiation which suppresses the body's defence mechanism.

Immunotherapy An experimental method of treatment that attempts to increase the body's own defence mechanisms against cancer.

Impotence Inability to engage in sexual intercourse. In men, impotence usually means the inability to experience an erection.

Incidence The rate at which a certain event occurs, such as the number of new cases of cancer occurring during a certain period.

Incisional Biopsy Surgical removal of part of a tissue to be examined.

In Situ Cancer The earliest stage of a cancer where it is localised just where it started.

Intravenous Pyelogram (IVP) Special test to check the urinary system involving X-rays and contrast dye.

Intravenous (IV) Infusion of fluid into a vein.

Irradiation Treatment by radiation.

Iscador An anthroposophic, homoeopathic preparation based on mistletoe, used for the destruction of cancer cells.

Laetrile The crystalline form of amygdalin.
Laparotomy An exploratory abdominal operation.
Laryngectomy Surgical removal of the voice box (larynx).
Laryngoscopy Examination of the back of the throat and voice box using a mirror.
Larynx Voice box, situated in the upper part of the wind pipe.
Lesion Any abnormal area (for whatever reason) in a tissue.
Leukaemia A cancer that originates in the blood-forming tissue of the bone marrow or the lymph nodes.
Leukocyte White blood cell.
Ley Line Line of energy in a landscape, often connecting churches or other community buildings, similar in action and therapeutic potential to the acupuncture meridians in the human body.
Libido Sexual desire.
Linear Accelerator A type of radiotherapy machine producing a very high energy radiation.
Localised Cancer A cancer confined to the site of origin.
Local Recurrence A tumour that reappears at the site of the original tumour.
Lumbar Puncture A test examining the fluid in the spine. After the area has been injected with local anaesthetic, a needle is inserted into the spine and fluid is taken out.
Lumpectomy (Tylectomy or Quadrantectomy) Surgical removal of a cancerous lump and a portion of surrounding tissue instead of the whole organ.
Lymphangiogram A special X-ray test to outline the lymph glands deep in the abdomen. A contrast dye is injected into the fine lymphatic vessels in the feet and this spreads to the abdomen.
Lymphatic System Circulatory network of lymph-carrying vessels, the lymph nodes, spleen, and thymus, which produce and store infection fighting cells.
Lymph Nodes Nodules of tissue in the lymphatic system that make lymphocytes and filter out unwanted substances.
Lymphocytes White cells in the blood that produce antibodies to fight infections.
Lymphoedema Swelling of a part of the body because the normal lymphatics have been blocked or destroyed.
Lymphoma A cancer that develops in the lymph system.
Macrobiotic Therapeutic dietary system based on organically-grown grains and fresh vegetables very simply cooked.
Macrophages Scavenger cells that bear away dead cells and other debris in the body.
Magnetic Resonance Scanning Measures the water content of tissue.
Mai or Mei or Mo In Chinese medicine, a meridian or channel in which body energies move, of which there are 12 principal ones.

Malignant A tumour which is cancerous.

Mammogram A special X-ray used to detect small breast cancers.

Mastectomy A surgical operation to remove a breast.

Mediastinum The part of the chest containing the heart and major blood vessels.

Mediastinoscopy A minor operation to look into the chest with a small telescope.

Medical Oncology The study of cancer.

Mega Voltage Radiotherapy High energy irradiation using cobalt or linear accelerator sources.

Mega Vitamin Therapeutic administration of high doses of vitamins.

Melanoma A cancer of the skin that develops from a mole.

Menarche The beginning of menstruation at puberty.

Menopause The cessation of menstruation.

Meridian See Mai. A channel of body energy which may be manipulated by the insertion of acupuncture needles into points along its course.

Mesothelioma A tumour of the lining of the lung (pleura) or of the abdomen (peritoneum) that is usually caused by contact with asbestos.

Metabolism The process by which the body's cells convert food to energy.

Metastasis The spread of cancer from one part of the body to another. The new area of cancer is a metastasis or secondary.

Metastatic Pathway The path travelled by cancerous cells when they spread from a tumour to distant parts of the body.

Micro Sievert Measure of radiation dose.

Mitosis The division by stages of a cell into two new cells.

Modulation The use of hypnosis and Biofeedback to make the brain cancel pain.

Molecule The smallest quantity into which a substance can be divided and still retain its characteristic properties.

Monocyte A large leucocyte with one nucleus.

Morbidity The symptoms or effects of a disease or its treatment.

Mortality Rate The death rate.

Mucositis Inflammation or soreness of the lining of the mouth (mucosa).

Mucous Membranes The lining tissue of such organs as the mouth and the intestine. By producing juices (secretions), the mucous membranes keep these organs moist.

Multicentric Having more than one centre of origin.

Mutation A change in the structure of a gene.

Mycotoxin Toxic substance found in fungal organisms.

Myeloma Cancer of the plasma cells in the bone marrow.

Myelogram A special test concerning the space around the spinal cord involving the use of X-rays and a contrast dye.

Nitrate In agricultural terminology, artificially-produced chemical fertiliser used to boost farm yields, but leading to lower-quality food and over-taxed soil.

Neoplasm Word sometimes used instead of cancer – it means new growth.

Neutrophils (Granulocytes) Infection-fighting cells in the blood.

Node Lymph node.

Nucleus The heart of a cell. The nucleus contains the genes.

Occult Tumour A hidden or concealed tumour.

Oedema Swelling caused by the accumulation of fluid in the body's tissues.

Oesophagus The tube connecting the mouth to the stomach – also known as the gullet.

Oestrogen A female hormone.

Oncology The study of tumours, both benign and malignant.

Oophorectomy (ovariectomy) A surgical operation to remove the ovaries.

Organic Having, or characterised by, organs; pertaining to living substances, as opposed to inorganic, non-living substances.

Orthodox Mainstream medical science, founded in a Cartesian or mechanistic view of the human being, whose principal therapeutic techniques are allopathic drug therapy and surgery.

Orthomolecular Study of the relationship between diet, health and disease.

Orthovoltage Radiotherapy Low energy radiation now used only to treat superficial cancers.

Osteopath Practitioner of a form of medicine in which the realignment of the bony skeleton, and thus the unlocking of patterns of muscular tension, improves the functioning of the whole person.

Ostomy The operation to form an artificial opening between an organ and the surface of the abdominal wall. This is done so that the excretion of the bowel, or urine, can be collected in a bag.

Paediatrician Specialist in child medicine.

Paget's Disease A cancer of the nipple.

Palliative Treatment Treatment aimed to kill pain or to make a person feel better rather than to cure.

Palpate Feel by hand.

PAP Smear See Cervical smear.

Paralytic Ileus Stoppage of the bowel caused by loss of normal intestinal movement.

Pathology Branch of medicine concerned with the study of disease; a state of disease.

Pectoralis Muscles The group of muscles on the front of the chest underlying the breast.

Peritoneum The inner lining of the abdomen.
Pharmacological Concerned with drugs and their action on the body.
Pituitary Gland The endocrine gland at the base of the brain which controls many other endocrine glands.
Placebo A harmless, ineffective substance given to a patient instead of a drug, often with a surprisingly high cure rate.
Platelets Cells in the blood that help it to clot.
Pleura The lining over the lungs.
Pleural Space Cavity between lungs and chest wall.
Polyp A benign outgrowth of tissue.
Polyunsaturated A class of mineral or vegetable fats consisting of long carbon chains with multiple bonds.
Pre-clinical Test Laboratory tests of a new drug or treatment. Pre-clinical tests must show that a drug or treatment is safe and effective before tests on human beings are allowed.
Pre-malignant An abnormal area in the body that may develop into a cancer but has not, as yet, done so.
Prevalence The total number of cases at one time in a given area.
Primary Cancer A cancer present at the site in which it developed.
Progesterone A hormone produced by the adrenal gland.
Prognosis A prediction of the likely course of a disease. This can be estimated only from the experiences of a lot of patients and cannot accurately predict the outcome for an individual.
Prolactin A pituitary hormone that stimulates milk production.
Prophylactic A treatment designed to prevent a disease.
Prostaglandin A group of essential fatty acids which affect the nervous system, circulation, female reproductive organs and metabolism.
Prostate A gland situated at the base of the bladder in front of the rectum in the male, which produces seminal fluid.
Prosthesis (Prosthetic device) A specially manufactured replacement to functionally and cosmetically take the place of a part of the body that has been surgically removed. The most common are artificial breasts after mastectomy and artificial limbs.
Protein A chemical containing, among other things, carbon, hydrogen, nitrogen and oxygen; an essential body nutrient.
Proteolytic Protein-digesting.
Protoplasm The material forming the essential substance of the living cell upon which life depends.
Psychotherapeutic Treatment using the mind and suggestion.
Psychosomatic Of mind and body, as in illness caused by emotions.
Quack From 'quacken' which is a mediaeval word for 'twitter'. A quackensalve was, therefore, one who twittered about his medicine, a charlatan.

Radiation The energy produced from radioactive substances, or from machines that emit X-rays.

Radiation Therapist (Radiotherapist) A doctor specialising in the treatment of cancer with radiation.

Radical Mastectomy An extensive mastectomy that includes removal of some of the muscles of the chest wall.

Radiesthesist Practitioner of a subtle form of medicine in which remedies, usually homoeopathic, are chosen and administered using the intuitive skill of a dowser.

Radioactive Implant The placing of a radioactive source in the body. This is put close to a cancer and gives it a very high dose of radiation and is then removed.

Radioactive Isotope A molecule that emits radiation.

Radiologist A doctor specialising in radioactive medicine such as X-rays.

Radionics Method of healing at a distance with the aid of extra sensory perception and specially designed instruments.

Radioresistant A tumour that does not shrink when treated with doses of radiation that can be tolerated by surrounding tissues.

Radiosensitive A cancer that shrinks or can be eradicated by a dose of radiation that is tolerated by nearby tissues.

Radiotherapy The treatment of cancer with X-rays.

Rate Radionics term for frequency of organs, diseases and remedies.

Reconstructive Mammaplasty The rebuilding of a breast by plastic surgery.

Registrar Middle-ranking hospital doctor.

Regression Returning to, or remembering, a former condition.

Relapse (Recurrence) The regrowth of a cancer after it has been removed or has responded to treatment.

Remission Shrinkage of a tumour. This may be partial or complete, but does not necessarily indicate cure.

Retro-Transportation Taking back from where it came.

Rubidium An alkali metal resembling potassium.

Sarcoma Cancer that develops in the body's supporting tissues (bone, cartilage, muscle, fat, tendons) and the tissue between organs.

Scanner An X-ray machine which systematically moves over a surface to examine it.

Secondary Tumour (Metastasis) A tumour that has developed in a distant part of the body as a result of cancerous cells having travelled from the site of the original cancer.

Selenium A trace element, deficiency of which can lead to impaired immune system and heart disease.

Sibling Brother or sister.

Side Effects Unwanted and sometimes unpleasant reactions to treatment that are usually temporary though some may be permanent.

Sigmoidoscopy A visual examination of the rectum and last part of the large bowel using a straight metal tube called a sigmoidoscope.

Simple Mastectomy (Total mastectomy) Surgical removal of the breast tissue only.

Staging The systematic investigation of the extent of spread of tumour in order to decide what treatment is best. The amount of tumour spread is described as the disease stage.

Steroids A group of naturally occurring compounds that may act as hormones, administered therapeutically for their action in reducing inflammation.

Stoma An opening in the flesh, formed by surgery, to allow for a body function that would otherwise be blocked.

Subcutaneous Mastectomy Surgical removal of the internal breast tissue, leaving the skin and nipple; used as a prophylactic measure.

Supraclavicular Relating to the area above the clavicle (collar bone). Usually used to refer to lymph nodes at this site.

Surgeon A doctor specialising in incisive medicine.

Surgery In relation to cancer, treatment in which cancerous tissue is removed from the body.

Surgical Oncologist A doctor specialising in cancer surgery.

Symptomatic Treatment Treatment that seeks to relieve a patient's symptoms, rather than to cure his disease.

Systemic Refers to the whole body: systemic treatment acts on the whole body.

Terminal The end; leading to death.

T-Lymphocytes White blood cells from the thymus gland.

Therapeutic Curative or healing.

Therapy Treatment for a disease.

Thermography Diagnosis by photographing the heat discharged by tissues. Infra-red radiation differs between normal and diseased tissue.

Thorascopy Examination of lungs by an instrument introduced through the chest.

Tissue Mass of cells of one kind.

Tomogram Special X-ray taken to find small abnormalities.

Toxic Poisonous.

Transcendental Rising above: a 'trade' name given to a specific form of meditation but generic to all meditation.

Transcutaneous Across the skin.

Tumour A swelling or mass of tissue in any part of the body. It may be cancerous or benign.

Tyelectomy (Lumpectomy) Surgical removal of a lump with a portion of surrounding tissue instead of the whole organ.

Ulcer An erosion in a surface membrane (such as in the stomach) that can be benign or malignant.

Ultrasound Test (Ultrasonography) The use of a very high frequency sound (which the ear cannot detect) to look inside the body.

Undifferentiated Cells Immature cells that are incapable of performing their proper function in the body. For example, an undifferentiated white blood cell cannot fight infection.

Urostomy The operation to form a new pathway made for the discharge of urine from the body.

Vaccine A substance injected into the body to create an immunity against a specific disease.

Venogram A special test to outline a vein, involving insertion of a fine catheter and use of contrast dye and X-rays.

Virus A small piece of genetic material encased in a coating of protein. Because it is a parasite, it can divide and multiply only when feeding on a living cell.

Vitamin An organic compound essential for the regulation of the metabolism.

White Blood Cells Cells that help the body to fight infection. White blood cells are produced in the bone marrow and the lymph nodes.

Witness Something associated with a patient, perhaps a hair, photograph or signature, used in place of their physical presence by a radiesthesist.

X-rays Highly active, invisible beams of energy.

Xeroradiograph A special X-ray of the breast.

Yang 'Sunny side of the mountain': positive, active, physical, scientific, masculine, hot.

Yin 'Shady side of the mountain': negative, cool, thoughtful, intuitive, receptive, feminine.

Useful Addresses

The following people will supply more detailed information on receipt of a stamped addressed envelope.

National Centres for Specialist Cancer Help and Information

Bacup, 121/123 Charterhouse Street, London EC1M 6AA. (01) 608 1661

Cancerlink, 46 Pentonville Road, London N1 9HF. (01) 833 2451

New Approaches to Cancer, c/o The Seekers Trust, Addington Park, Maidstone, Kent ME19 5BL. (0732) 848336

Complementary

Anthroposophical Medical Association, Rudolf Steiner House, 35 Park Road, London NW1. (01) 723 4400

Association for Humanistic Psychology in Britain, 5 Layton Road, London N1. (01) 226 4240

Association of Hypnotists and Psychotherapists, 25 Market Square, Nelson, Lancs. (0282) 699378

Dr Edward Bach Centre, Mount Vernon, Sotwell, Oxon OX10 OPZ. (0491) 39489

British Association of Art Therapists, 88 Bridport Close, Lower Earley, Reading.

British Homoeopathic Association, 27a Devonshire Street, London W1N 1RJ. (01) 935 2163

British Medical Acupuncture Society, 67/69 Chancery Lane, London WC2A 1AF.

British Naturopathic and Osteopathic Association, 6 Netherall Gardens, London NW3 5RR. (01) 435 7830

British Society for Medical and Dental Hypnosis, PO Box 6, 42 Links Road, Ashtead, Surrey KT21 2HJ.

British Society for Music Therapy, 69 Avondale Avenue, East Barnet, Herts EN4 8NB.

British Wheel of Yoga, General Secretary, 80 Lechampton Road, Cheltenham, Glos.

Centre for Transpersonal Psychology, 7 Pembridge Place, London W2 4XB.

Colour Therapy, Aura Soma, Chilton House, Gold Hill West, Chalfont St Peter, Bucks SL9 9HH. (0753) 886840.

Council for Acupuncture, 10 Belgrave Square, London SW1X 8PH.

East-West Foundation, 188 Old Street, London EC1.

Harry Edwards Healing Sanctuary, Burrows Lea, Shere, Guildford, Surrey. (048641) 2054 Organises contact and absent healing.

Friends of Shanti Nilaya, PO Box 212, London NW8 7NW. Aims to provide support based on the work of Dr Elizabeth Kubler Ross.

Institute for Complementary Medicine, 21 Portland Place, London W1N 3AF. (01) 636 9543 Public information and documentation service. Will supply name and address of local practitioner in chiropractic, acupuncture, osteopathy, medical herbalism and homoeopathy: will supply the national addresses of the remaining complementary specialities.

Institute of Psychosynthesis, 1 Cambridge Gate, Regent's Park, London NW1 4JN. (01) 486 2588

Matthew Manning Centre, 39 Abbeygate Street, Bury St Edmunds, Suffolk IP33 1LW. (0284) 69502/2364

National Council and Register of Iridology, 80 Portland Road, Bournemouth, Dorset BH9 1NQ. (0202) 529793

National Federation of Spiritual Healers, Old Manor Farm Studio, Sunbury-on-Thames, Middx TW16 6RG. (09327) 83164

National Institute of Medical Herbalists, Secretary: PO Box 3, 41 Hatherley Road, Winchester, Hants SO22 6RR. (0962) 68776

Register of British Acupuncturists, 34 Alderney Street, London SW1V 4EU. (01) 854 1012

Register of Osteopaths, 21 Suffolk Street, London SW1Y 4HG. (01) 839 2060

Radionics Association, 16a North Bar, Banbury, Oxfordshire OX16 0TF. (0295) 3183

Royal London Homoeopathic Hospital, Great Ormond Street, London WC1 3HC. (01) 837 3091

Society of Homoeopaths, 11a Bampton Street, Tiverton, Devon EX16 6HH. (0884) 255117

Society of Teachers of the Alexander Technique, 10 London House, 266 Fulham Road, London SW10 9EL. (01) 351 0828 The Alexander Technique is a method of redeploying every part of the body to work efficiently and so to prevent or cure a wide range of physical and mental disorders.

A Selection of Cancer Centres

Contact Cancerlink or New Approaches to Cancer for your nearest help point.

Auchenkyle Health Centre, South Wood Road, Troon, Ayrshire. (0292) 311414

Bournemouth Centre of Complementary Medicine, 26 Sea Road, Boscombe, Bournemouth, Dorset BH5 1DF. (0202) 36354

Bristol Cancer Help Centre, Grove House, Cornwallis Grove, Bristol BS8 4PG. (0272) 743216

The Contreras Clinic, Clinico del Mar, Tijuana, Mexico.

CYANA, 31 Church Road, London E12 6AD. (01) 533 5366

The Gerson Institute, PO Box 430, Bonita, California 92002, USA.

Dr Josef Issels, The RingbergKlinic, Bad Wiessee, Bavaria.

Morecambe Bay Cancer Help Centre, Secretary: Mrs Janet Stewart, 11 College Road, Windermere, Cumbria LA23 1BU. (09662) 2548

Park Attwood Centre, Trimbley, Bewdley, Worcs DY12 1RE. (02997) 444

Ms Margaret Straus, 87 Via Nazionale, 22050-Colico (Coma) Italy.

Wessex Cancer Help Centre, 8 South Street, Chichester, West Sussex PO19 1EH. (0243) 778516

Children

Centre for Attitudinal Healing, PO Box 638, London SW3 4LN. (01) 235 6733

Children's Cancer Help Centre, 51 Woodcote Drive, Orpington, Kent BR6 8DR.

Mrs Bernadette Cleary, Dove Cottage Self Help Group, 16 The Glade, Fetcham, Leatherhead, Surrey KT22 9TH.

National Association for the Welfare of Children in Hospital, Argyle House, 29–31 Euston Road, London NW1 2SD. (01) 833 2041

Malcolm Sargent Cancer Fund for Children, 14 Abingdon Road, London W8 6AF. (01) 937 4548

Nutrition

Henry Doubleday Research Association, National Centre for Organic Gardening, Ryton-on-Dunsmore, Coventry CV8 3LG. (0203) 303517

Laetrile, Leon Chaitow, c/o Thorsons Publishers, Denington Estate, Wellingborough, Northants.

Macrobiotics, Community Health Foundation, 188 Old Street, London EC1V 9BP. (01) 251 4076

Organic Growers Association, Aeron Park, Llangeitho, Dyfed, Wales. (0272) 299800

Soil Association, 86 Colston Street, Bristol BS1 5BB. (0272) 290661

Vegan Society, 33–35 George Street, Oxford OX1 2AY.

Vegetarian Society, 53 Marloes Road, London W8 6LA. (01) 937 7739

Practical Help

Association of Carers, 1st Floor, 21–23 New Road, Chatham, Kent ME4 4QJ. National organisation, offering support to relatives, the chronically ill or disabled and giving practical advice plus contacts for local self-help groups.

Brighton Cancer Prevention Foundation, 6 New Road, Brighton, Sussex. (0273) 727213

British Red Cross Society, 9 Grosvenor Crescent, London SW1X 7EJ. (01) 235 5454

Brook Advisory Centre, 153a East Street, London SE17 2ED. (01) 708 1234 Centres also in Birmingham, Bristol, Coventry, Edinburgh and Liverpool.

BUPA, Provident House, Essex Street, London WC2R 3AX. (01) 353 5212

Family Planning Association, 27/35 Mortimer Street, London W1N 7RJ. (01) 636 7866

Institute for Sex Education Research, 40 School Road, Birmingham. (021) 4490892

Lisa Sainsbury Foundation, 8–10 Crown Hill, Croydon, Surrey CR0 1RY. (01) 686 8809

Macmillan Nurses, c/o The National Society for Cancer Relief, Anchor House, 15–19 Britten Street, London SW3 3TY. (01) 351 7811

Marie Curie Memorial Foundation, 28 Belgrave Square, London SW1 (01) 235 3325

National Consumer Council, Grosvenor Gardens, London SW1.

Private Patients Plan, PPP House, Crescent Road, Tunbridge Wells, Kent TN1 2PL. (0892) 40111

Psychosexual Unit, Mandsley Hospital, Denmark Hill, London SE5 8A2. (01) 703 6333

Organisations Giving Help/Information on Specific Cancers

Action on Smoking and Health, 5–11 Mortimer Street, London W1N 7RH. (01) 637 9843

Chest, Heart and Stroke Association, Tavistock House North, Tavistock Square, London WC1H 9JE. (01) 387 3012 Gives financial aid and counselling to people with lung cancer.

Colostomy Welfare Group, 38/39 Eccleston Square, London SW1V 1PB. (01) 828 5175 The aim is to help the mental, spiritual and physical adjustment of those who have had, or are about to have, a colostomy. They place importance on home and hospital visiting.

Ileostomy Association of GB and Ireland, Amblehurst House, Chobham, Woking, Surrey GU24 8PZ. (09905) 8277

Let's Face It, 10 Woodend, Crowthorne, Berks. (0344) 774405

Leukaemia Care Society, PO Box 82, Exeter, Devon EX2 5DP. (0392) 218514

Leukaemia Research Fund, 43 Great Ormond Street, London WC1N 3JJ. (01) 405 0101 Produces a series of booklets about leukaemia and other disorders.

Mastectomy Association of Great Britain, 26 Harrison Street, Off Grays Inn Road, Kings Cross, London WC1H 8JG. (01) 837 0908

National Association of Laryngectomee Clubs, 4th Floor, 39 Eccleston Square, London SW1V 1PB. (01) 834 2857

Society for the Prevention of Asbestiosis and Industrial Diseases, 39 Drapers Road, Enfield, Middx EN2 8LU. (01) 366 1640

Stoma Advisory Service, Abbott Laboratories Ltd, Queenborough, Kent ME11 5EL. (0795) 663371 Although run by a manufacturer, this group will provide independent advice and also publishes useful booklets.

Urostomy Association, Mrs Angela Cooke, Buckland, Beaumont Park, Danbury, Essex CM3 4DE. Provides information for patients who have had a urinary diversion.

Women's National Cancer Control Campaign, 1 South Audley Street, London W1Y 5DQ. (01) 499 7532 WNCCC centres also in Warrington, Macclesfield, Harrogate, Berkhamstead, Luton, Brighton, Maidstone, Cleveland, Aberdeen, Cardiff and Camberwell.

Official Bodies

British Holistic Medical Association, 179 Gloucester Place, London NW1 6DX. (01) 262 5299

British Medical Association, Tavistock Square, London WC1H 9JP. (01) 387 4499

College of Health, 18 Victoria Park Square, Bethnal Green, London E2 9PF.

Department of Health and Social Security, Alexander Fleming House, Elephant and Castle, London SE1 6BY. (01) 407 5522

Government department responsible for central planning of the NHS and for monitoring its performance.

National Radiological Protection Board, Chilton, Didcot, Oxfordshire OX11 9RQ. Abingdon (0235) 831600

Hospice

Hospice Information, St Christopher's Hospice, 51/59 Lawrie Park, Sydenham, London SE26 6DZ. (01) 778 9252 Information about all hospice and domiciliary services, and an extensive book list on related subjects.

St Joseph's Hospice, Mare Street, Hackney, London E8. (01) 985 0861 A working hospice, dealing particularly with cancer patients. Has a list of hospices elsewhere in the UK.

Short-stay Residential Centres

Burrswood, Groombridge, Tunbridge Wells, Kent. A medical healing centre in beautiful grounds.

Claridge House, Dormansland, Lingfield, Surrey. Vegetarian.

Harmony House, Southerton, Ottery St Mary, Devon. (0395) 68946 A holistic vegetarian guest-house.

Charities and Research

British Association for the Advancement of Science, 23 Savile Row, London W1. (01) 734 6010 For copies of academic papers on latest cancer research.

Cancer Research Campaign, 2 Carlton House Terrace, London SW1Y 5AR. (01) 930 8972

Charities Aid Foundation, 48 Pembury Road, Tonbridge, Kent TN9 2JD. (0732) 356323 Organisation set up specifically to help and co-ordinate the raising and distribution of funds to charities.

Imperial Cancer Research, Lincolns Inn Field, PO Box 123, London WC2A 3PX. (01) 242 0200

Marie Curie Memorial Foundation, 28 Belgrave Square, London SW1X 8QG. (01) 235 3325

National Society for Cancer Relief, Anchor House, 15–19 Britten Street, London SW3 3TY. (01) 351 7811

Richard Dimbleby Cancer Fund, St Thomas's Hospital, Lambeth Palace Road, London SE1. Raises funds for St Thomas's Hospital and other cancer charities.

Royal Marsden Hospital, Patient Education Group, Fulham Road, London SW3 6JJ. (01) 352 8171 ext. 437

Sue Ryder Foundation, Cavendish, Nr Sudbury, Suffolk. Glemsford (0787) 280252

Wallace Kingston Trust for Abdominal Diseases, The Drove, Fuzzy Drove, Basingstoke, Hants. (0256) 52320 Has a residential home in Leeds with seventeen beds.

World Federation for Cancer Care, 28 Belgrave Square, London SW1X 8QG. (01) 235 3325 Gives information on all contacts worldwide.

Other Help

Animal Health Trust, Landways Hall, Newmarket, Suffolk (0638) 751 030 Trust Headquarters and centre for small animals.

Animal Health Trust, PO Box 5, Balaton Lodge, Snailwell Road, Newmarket, Suffolk CB8 7DW. (0638) 661111 For horses.

The British Fluoridation Society, 63 Wimpole Street, London W1M 8AL.

British Humanist Association, 13 Prince of Wales Terrace, London W8 5PG. (01) 937 2341

Churches Council for Health and Healing, St Marylebone Parish Church, Marylebone Road, London NW1 5LT. (01) 935 7315 Interdenominational organisation representing British Churches and allied professions 'for mutual consultation and cooperative action.'

Ecoropa UK Ltd, Henbant Fach, Llanbedr, Crickhowell, Powys, Wales. (0873) 810758 Ecological Action Group for Europe: for information and leaflets on cancer prevention, nutrition, additives/ diet.

National Consumer Council, Grosvenor Gardens, London SW1. (01) 222 9501.

National Pure Water Association, Bank Farm, Aston Pigott, Westbury, Shrewsbury, SY5 9HH. Worthen (074 383) 445.

Further Reading

The book list could be endless. Here are a few titles that may help you in the next stage of your quest:

A Cancer Therapy – the results of 50 cases, Max Gerson (Totality Books, Del Mar)
A Reckoning, May Sarton (Women's Press)
A Time to Heal, Beata Bishop (Severn House, 1985)
About Laetrile, Leon Chaitow (Thorsons, 1979)
Additives – Your Complete Survival Guide, Ed. by Felicity Lawrence (Century, 1986)
All About Cancer, Chris Williams (John Wiley & Sons, 1984)
An End to Cancer – A Nutritional Approach to Cancer and its Cure, Leon Chaitow (Thorsons, 1978)
Anatomy of an Illness, Norman Cousins (Bantam, 1981)
Cancer – A Guide for Patients and their Families, Chris & Sue Williams (John Wiley & Sons, 1986)
Cancer and Diet (The Commuity Foundation)
Cancer in Britain – the Politics of Prevention, Lesley Doyal & Sue Epstein (Pluto Press)
Cancer Myths and Realities, Dr L. Kothari & L. Mehtha (Marion Boyars, 1979)
Charities Aid Foundation Directory of Cancer Research and Welfare Organisations (Charities Aid Foundation)
Choices, Marion Morra & Eve Potts (Avon Books, New York, 1980)
Contrary to Nature, Michael B. Shumkin (US Dept of Health, 1979)
Death and Dying, Elizabeth Kubler Ross (Shanti Nilaya, UK)
Facing Death, Diana Lampen (Quaker Home Service, 1979)
Fighting for Our Lives, Kit Mouat (Heretic Books)
Gentle Giants, Penny Brohn (Century, 1986)
Getting Well Again, Carl Simonton (Bantam Books, USA, 1978)
How to Avoid Cancer, Dr Jan de Winter (Dr Jan de Winter, 1981)
How to Live Longer and Feel Better, Dr Linus Pauling (W. H. Freeman)
How to Meditate, Le Shan (Turnstone Press)

Making the Vitamin Connection, James Scala, PhD (Harper & Row, New York, 1980)

Mind as Healer Mind as Slayer, Kenneth R. Pelletier (New York, 1977)

New Hope and Improved Treatment for Cancer Patients, David Holmes (David Holmes, 1982)

Patients' Guide to the National Health (Consumer Council)

Patients' Rights (National Consumer Council, 1983)

Prevention and Cure of Cancer, Julhim A. Hassan (Exposition Press, USA, 1983)

The Ageing Factor, Dr John Yiamouyannis (Health Action Press, 1983)

The Alternative Health Guide, Brian Inglis & Ruth West (Michael Joseph, 1983)

The Atlas of Cancer Mortality, M. J. Gardner (Wiley)

The BUPA Manual of Fitness and Wellbeing (Macdonald, 1984)

The Cancer Prevention Diet – Macrobiotics, Ed. by Edward Esko (East West Foundation, 1981)

The Cancer Reference Book, Paul M. Levitt & Elissa S. Guranick (Paddington Press, 1979)

The Causes of Cancer, Dr R. Doll & Dr A. Peto (OUP)

The Christian Agnostic, Lesley Weatherhead (Hodder & Stoughton)

The Death of Ivan Illych, Leo Tolstoy (Bradder Books, distr. by Basil Blackwell)

The Diseases of Civilisation, Brian Inglis (Hodder & Stoughton, 1981)

The Doctor's Dilemma, George Bernard Shaw (1911)

The Gate of Healing, Ian Pearce (Jersey Neville Spearman, 1983)

The Healing Family, Stephanie Matthews Simonton (Bantam, 1984)

The Holistic Approach to Cancer, Dr. Ian Pearce (ANAC, 1980)

The Holistic Herbal, David Hoffman (Findhorn Press)

The Hospice Movement, Sandol Stoddard (Jonathan Cape, 1979)

The Medical Discoveries of Edward Bach, Physician, Norah Weeks (The G. W. Daniel Co., 1983)

The Positive Health Guide (Martin Dunitz)

The Power to Heal, David Harvey (The Aquarian Press, 1983)

The Siege of Cancer, June Goodfield (Random House, New York, 1975)

The Topic of Cancer, Dick Richards (Pergamon Press, 1982)

The Turning Point, Frijof Capra (Fontana)

The Wayward Cell: Cancer, Victor Richards (Berkeley, California, 1978)

There is a Rainbow Behind Every Dark Cloud (selection of children's art) (Centre for Attitudinal Healing, California, 1979)

You Can Fight for Your Life, Lawrence le Shan (Thorsons, 1980)

Index